BIOETHICAL DILEMMAS IN HEALTH OCCUPATIONS

BIOETHICAL DILEMMAS IN HEALTH OCCUPATIONS

Margaret Snell, Editor

GLENCOE
Macmillan / McGraw-Hill

Lake Forest, Illinois
Columbus, Ohio
Mission Hills, California
Peoria, Illinois

Copyright (c) 1991 by the Glencoe Division of Macmillan/McGraw-Hill Publishing Company. All rights reserved. Printed in the United States of America. Except as permitted under the United States Copyright Act of 1976, no part of this publication may be reproduced or distributed in any form or by any means, or stored in a database or retrieval system, without prior permission of the publisher.

Send all inquiries to:
Glencoe Division, Macmillan/McGraw-Hill
809 West Detweiller Dr.
Peoria, IL 61615-2190

ISBN 0-02-685650-6

1 2 3 4 5 6 7 8 9   94 93 92 91 90

TABLE OF CONTENTS

8   Eugenics: Should Human Hereditary Traits Be Enhanced?
    Karen E. Gable

20 Splicing Genes to Understand, Interpret, and Change Nature
    Paul Hoeksema

32 Patient Selection in Kidney Dialysis
    Patricia Kearns Leitsch

44 In-Vitro Fertilization, Embryo Transfer, and Surrogate Mothers
    Mary Lou Park

58 Human Behavior Control: Realities and Possibilities
    Ruth M. Patterson

68 Fetal Research
    Mildred M. Pittman

76 Mass Screening for Genetic Disorders
    Mildred M. Pittman

90 Issues and Problems of Organ Transplantation
    Janice R. Sandiford

100 Scientific Knowledge Versus Human Experimentation
    Norma Jean Schira

110 Medicine's Chaos: The Terminally Ill
    Margaret Snell

126 Infanticide: An Ethical Dilemma
    Norma J. Walters

142 Photo Credits

143 Index

Chapter Scenarios were written by Arlene Morris and Margaret Snell

Introduction

Any textbook that purports to discuss a continually changing subject such as medical bioethics is doomed to failure before it is ever published unless readers understand that the primary purpose of the text is to provide students with an opportunity to examine their bioethical values. Associated with that purpose are the related needs for students to understand some of the variables that influence bioethical decision making and to become cognizant of the value systems of other people. Students who plan to work in the health care field, in particular, should have an opportunity to examine their feelings regarding bioethical concerns before being confronted with the emotions inherent in an actual situation, whether it is one that impacts directly on their personal life or one in which they are an interested, empathetic bystander. Students should know and be able to accept their bioethical value systems, and be comfortable with any bioethical decisions they might have to make.

The need for students to experience this type of learning was expressed at a planning session for a national convention which would be attended by classroom teachers, state supervisors, and college professors, specifically the Health Occupations Education division of the American Vocational Association. After discussion it was decided to present a bioethics program and to utilize the expertise of the membership. The resulting program was well attended and enthusiastically received.

Because of the widespread interest generated by that program a text was envisioned that would parallel the symposium. Therefore, the subjects selected for this text reflect the topics presented at that national convention.

Each chapter has two scenarios associated with the topic: one short situation that can be resolved without extensive discussion and one long situation that involves a number of decisions. There are no "right" answers. The scenarios are included to enable students to review their thinking on bioethical issues and to become aware of their peers' thinking via discussion of the scenarios.

The terminology at the beginning of each chapter includes terms suggested by students in a health occupations program offered at Willingboro High School, New Jersey, an average middle-class community in a suburban/rural area of the state. By defining the terms identified by those students as needing some explanation, it is expected that the text will be useful for students in high school through graduate level programs. Certainly the scenarios can be discussed at different levels depending upon students' knowledge and background

Today's students will become tomorrow's decision makers. The ever-increasing advances in medical technology present an awesome responsibility in situations where there are no "right" answers, only choices that hopefully will become valid and just decisions. This text, offering an overview of medical bioethical issues with the accompanying scenarios, is designed to stimulate students' interest in the topics and to assist future decision makers to function as effectively as possible in our ever-changing world.

1

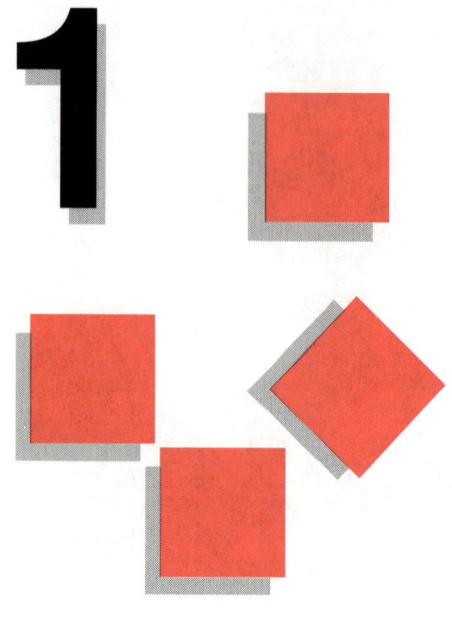

Eugenics: Should Human Hereditary Traits Be Enhanced?

by Karen E. Gable*

Objectives

After reading this chapter, you should be able to:
- Define the terms listed at the beginning of this chapter.
- Define **eugenics** in your own words.
- Differentiate between **negative eugenics** and **positive eugenics.**
- Identify the two historical periods of the eugenics movement in the United States.
- Explain at least three different perspectives of the eugenics issue.
- Make a personal decision about the use of eugenics.
- Defend a personal position on the issue.

Terms and Definitions

Contraception. Prevention of conception.
Defective genes. Hereditary units that are imperfect.
DNA probes. DNA (deoxyribonucleic acid) fragments used in genetic studies.
Eugenics. The study of hereditary improvements, especially of human improvement, by genetic control.
Fecundity. The capability of producing young in abundance.
Gametes. Mature sperm or egg cells that are capable of participating in fertilization.
Genetic engineering. The use of technology to manipulate genes.
In-vitro fertilization. The process of initiating reproduction in an artificial environment such as a test tube.
Negative eugenics. Hereditary improvement by elimination of inferior traits.
Positive eugenics. Hereditary improvement by enhancement of superior traits.
Prenatal screening. Testing which is done before birth of a baby.

Introduction

Eugenics, the study of hereditary improvement, has emerged in the 1980s as an issue involving the health care industry and society as a whole. New techniques such as **in vitro fertilization** and **prenatal screening for genetic disorders** are having an impact on the process of reproduction and on who gets born: more infertile couples can now bear children, and more fertile ones can abort fetuses that are known to carry such inherited disorders as Down's syndrome. With the recent development of some sophisticated new scientific procedures, known collectively as **genetic engineering** or **gene therapy**, manipulating heredity through gene control is soon to become a reality. But how should this new technology be applied? And should it even *be* applied?

- Is it moral for humans to interfere with a natural biological process as reproduction?
- Will gene control be used altruistically, e.g., to reduce the incidence of inherited diseases?
- Is there a danger that gene control will be used to weed out particular groups or races as "undesirable"?
- Is it ethical to tamper with an embryo?

Even before these recent advances occurred, the makeup of a population was sometimes manipulated in other ways. Perhaps the most notorious example was the Nazi genocide of the Jews to purify the German race. Sterilization has been used to prevent reproduction, and legislation has been enacted to restrict the entry of certain immigrant groups into a nation.

To better understand the complex issue of eugenics, we can look at it from several perspectives:

- political/legal
- economic
- social
- scientific
- philosophical/moral/ethical

These perspectives affect decision making at the personal, social, and political levels. In the final analysis, it is the citizenry, as individuals and as a collective body, who must resolve the questions and issues related to eugenics and their implications for society.

According to Melendy (1904, p. i),

The goal of eugenics is the betterment of the human race, and it embraces all forces and factors, whether hygienic, biological, social, or economic, which are, or may be, influential in the uplifting and improvement of mankind.... It is the aim of eugenics to conserve the higher elements of human heredity so that each succeeding generation will be able to realize a larger balance on the side of normal mentality, strong physique, and high moral attainment. The eugenic vision is the elimination of the limits and risks in natural human reproduction.

---

*Karen E. Gable
Assistant Professor of Health Occupations Education,
Indiana University, Indianapolis, Indiana.

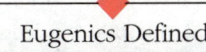
Eugenics Defined

The improvement of the stock, which is by no means confined to questions of judicious mating but, which, especially in the case of man (sic), takes cognizance of all the influences that tend in however remote a degree to give the more suitable races or strains of blood a better chance of prevailing speedily over the less suitable than they otherwise would have had.

Hubbard (1986, p. 229)

"... the movement to improve and even perfect the human species by technological means..."

Neuhaus (1988)

Eugenics Movement Around the World

The eugenics movement has been active in several countries throughout the world during various periods. The British eugenics movement developed during the latter part of the nineteenth and the early twentieth centuries and continued to count many prominent biologists and social scientists among its supporters in the 1930s and 1940s. As late as 1941, Julian Huxley, the eminent biologist, wrote the article "The Vital Importance of Eugenics." His opening words were prophetic — "Eugenics . . . has ceased to be regarded as a fad . . . and in the near future will be regarded as an urgent practical matter."

The German movement, probably the most infamous, sought in the 1930s and 1940s to improve the race of German people by ridding it of inferior and foreign elements. The German "racial hygiene" eugenics movement was founded in 1895 and addressed the same three social fears or problems as that in Britain:

- Humane care for people with disabilities would enfeeble the "race" because they would survive to pass their disabilities on to their children.

- Not just mental and physical diseases and so-called defects but also poverty, criminality, alcoholism, prostitution, and other social problems were based in biology and inherited.

- Genetically inferior people were reproducing faster than superior people and would eventually displace them.

Recently, Singapore has implemented policies related to eugenics. In August of 1983, the Prime Minister stressed the importance of producing quality persons who would be able to sustain Singapore's economic growth. Believing that the fate of Singapore rests with an elite group who possesses greater physical and mental aptitudes than the common person, the government has established policies that carry over into social and educational activities. An elaborate and complex system of tracking students in the educational system is one method used to identify potential members of the elite group. Incentives (money and education) are offered to women who are graduates of the system to bear more children. Computer dating services and all expense paid "love-boat" cruises for eligible singles are elements of the government package to encourage the educated to bear children.

A complimentary measure aimed at less-educated women was instituted as well. Rewards of a down-payment (equivalent of $4,000 in U.S. dollars) were given to women who were less than 30 years of age, had two or fewer children, had an educational level not beyond the junior high level, and were willing to be sterilized.

Confronted with a very large population and widespread poverty, government leadership in China has been concerned about population growth and its implications for the future. State-mandated contraception and abortion, official encouragement of late marriages, and economic and social sanctions against couples who have several children are efforts that have been tried.

In the United States, the eugenics movement had the greatest influence during two historical periods: 1905-25 and 1950-60s. During the initial period, more than half of the states in America had mandatory sterilization laws which were applied to people who fell into the described categories of the unfit such as the feebleminded.

The 1950s and the 1960s reflected a renewed interest in eugenic problems, but the period lacked the scientific knowledge, technology, and general supportive social attitudes to achieve significance. In the 1980s, interest redeveloped in old and new eugenic problems. Major advances in scientific knowledge and technological innovations have created many questions related to eugenics.

Galton

Francis Galton coined the term eugenics in 1883. The word eugenics is derived from the Greek word for "wellborn." Galton was born in England in 1822 of parents who strongly wanted him to be a doctor as were his mother's father and stepbrother. He began his apprenticeship in 1836 at Birmingham General Hospital but abandoned all thought of becoming a doctor after his father's death in 1844. By 1900, Galton had decided that the improvement of the human race could be placed on a scientific basis.

"Eugenics" (a term which he created) became his obsession. He funded a laboratory and bequeathed money to the University of London for the study of eugenics. Just three years before his death in 1911, Galton published *Memories of My Life* which relates his experiences as a medical student as well as suggests ways of improving the practice of medicine.

The underlying concern of the American movement is represented by Lewis Terman, a proponent for IQ testing: "The fecundity of the family stocks from which our most gifted children come appears to be definitely on the wane," (Hubbard, 1986, p. 230). To tackle this problem, the movement launched a two-fold program:

- **positive eugenics:** encouraging the "fit" (read "well-to-do") to have lots of children.

- **negative eugenics:** preventing the "unfit" (defined to include people suffering from insanity, epilepsy, alcoholism, "pauperism," criminality, "sexual perversion," drug abuse, and especially "feeblemindedness") from having any children.

The 1980s and 1990s are becoming the third period. Many recently developed advanced technologies have applications in the health care fields.

Multiple Perspectives on Eugenics

Like any complex issue or situation, eugenics can be viewed from multiple perspectives. The perspectives covered here are: political/legal, social, scientific, and philosophical/moral/ethical.

Political/Legal: Governmental Manipulation of the Population Mix

The political perspective is represented by the utilization of the negative eugenics approach (i.e., genocide) by the notorious Nazi Germany government and the recent calls for "positive eugenics . . . to accelerate the birth of individuals possessing outstanding physical and intellectual qualities" in Singapore (Chan, 1985, p. 707).

In the United States, a vocal minority in the 1920s and 1930s was successful in promoting legislation for the restriction of immigrants. By limiting the number of immigrants to reflect the percentages in the 1890 census, the 1924 Immigration Restriction Act decreased the proportion of poor immigrants from southern and eastern Europe and gave preference to immigrants from Britain and Northern Europe.

Both state and federal governments have enacted laws dealing with eugenics. States have enacted laws that have claimed for themselves the right to decide who should inhabit their territory. Sterilization acts were aimed primarily at the insane, feebleminded, perverts, drug addicts, drunkards, epileptics, and any other diseased or degenerate persons. States passed legislation prohibiting interracial marriage until the U.S. Supreme Court declared that this was in violation of the Fourteenth Amendment.

Economic: Expenses Connected with Heredity

One example of the economic perspective is concern for the expenses to parents and society of raising disabled children. The costs of meeting the special needs of people with inherited disorders such as Down's syndrome and spina bifida may be astronomical and continue over a lifetime. The reimbursement policies of federal agencies for fertility treatment and genetic therapy have also been an element of the economic perspective.

Social: The Relationship of Heredity and Social Problems

The eugenics movement grew in response to the fear that social problems such as poverty, criminality, alcoholism, and prostitution were based in biology and inherited. The relationship of heredity and social problems has been researched and debated. Sociologists express concern that a simplistic approach to the cause of social problems may be unfounded. Some members of society believe that immigration can or will cause degeneration of the native population.

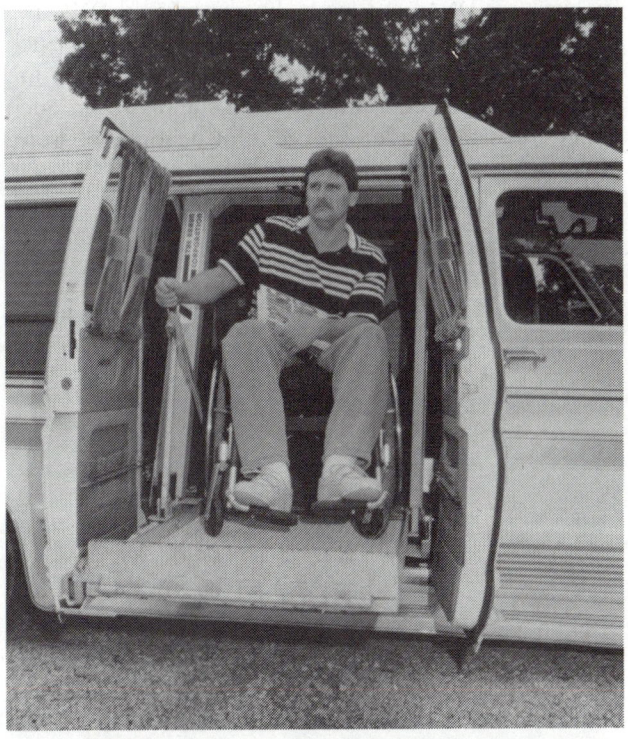

Will the public always be willing to provide the funds for services for persons with disabilities?

Scientific: Genetic Inferiority and Superiority

Biologists and those persons who address eugenics from a scientific perspective have suggested that the eugenics movement responded to the fear that prolonging the lives of people with disabilities would dilute the "race" because the disabled would pass their disabilities on to their children. In addition, people deemed genetically inferior were believed to be reproducing faster than superior people and might eventually displace them. The eugenics measures have been and are regarded as health measures from a scientific perspective.

Relevant scientific efforts in molecular DNA research involve identifying genetic problems and ultimately finding solutions to those problems.

Defective genes related to conditions such as Down's syndrome, sickle-cell anemia, hemophilia, and muscular dystrophy can be identified. The use of **DNA probes**, fragments of DNA, provides information about the genetic makeup of an organism.

Today tests can detect neural tube developmental defects (NTDs). The usefulness of such tests is still somewhat questionable because of a high rate of false-positive results and because they cannot indicate the severity of the deformity. Such tests will continue, however, to be developed and improved.

It is now possible to isolate a single gene from an organism's total DNA, recombine it with a carrier molecule or DNA, and insert the recombined DNA into an infected cell to produce a modified organism. Such molecular techniques are currently used to study the relationship between viral infections and cancer. Such procedures fall under the general heading of **gene therapy** or **genetic engineering.** It is already possible to replace a defective gene with a normal one.

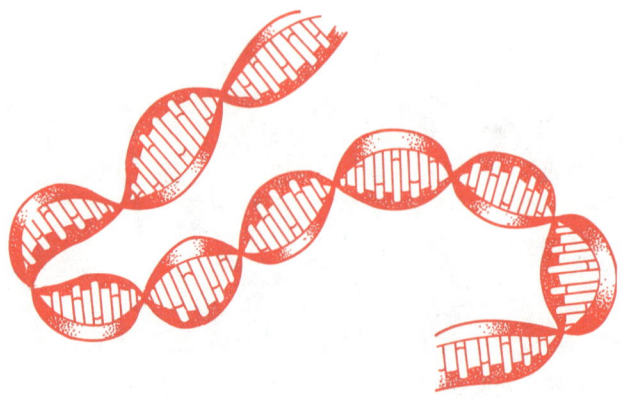

Philosophical/Moral/Ethical: Considering the Basic Issue

The philosophical perspective concerns the value systems by which society exists. Analysis and critique of the formulation and development of personal and societal beliefs have lead to many questions.

Some of the philosophical questions considered are:

- What is the value of living when faced with the potential of becoming sick and dying at some unknown future date, e.g., in the person's thirties, forties, or fifties?
- What is the relationship between the collective body of people and the rights of the individual?
- Should gene therapy be the exclusive or primary way to eliminate or reduce genetic problems?

The philosophical perspective has been used as the basis for the position that the "fit" should inhabit the world as well as for making decisions on the application of advanced technologies. Philosophical viewpoints may differ because of varying religious and ideological values.

Many persons, organizations, and institutions have attempted to address the issue of eugenics from ethical and moral viewpoints. Concern has been expressed over the ethics involved in tampering with an embryo (Chomsky, 1983; Talbot, 1983), the multiple questions related to the applications of scientific developments (Chomsky, 1983), and the moral responsibility of individuals to consider the quality of life for unborn generations. Efforts of the national government to address ethical issues have led to the written recommendations of the 1983 President's Commission for the Study of Ethical Problems in Medicine and Biomedical and Behavioral Research (Merz, 1984), and to Congress addressing the ethical issues of genetic engineering (Wallace, 1984). Five basic recommendations were included in the Commission's report:

1. Genetic information should not be made available to persons unrelated to the client except in adoption cases when serious genetic risks should be communicated to the adoptive parents of adopted children.
2. Mandatory screening is justified only when voluntary procedures are inadequate to prevent harm to defenseless persons such as children.
3. Disclosure should be presumed in deliberations regarding the release of incidental findings such as might occur in paternity cases.
4. Screening programs should only be initiated after thorough study of the testing procedures has occurred.

5. Availability and access to screening should recognize the rates of incidence of genetic disorders in various ethnic and racial groups without being discriminatory.

These guidelines hopefully will protect individual rights in public screenings. However, they probably will not have major influence upon private industry. Genetic information could pose a problem for people at risk for early death. Insurance companies might use such information to deny insurance coverage. Likewise, employment could be denied to persons for whom working conditions pose a risk.

A central question for discussion of moral and ethical aspects of genetic screening and therapy is who — the affected individual, private industry, or government — should determine which people will undergo the testing.

Ethical concerns focus on the major questions of:

Who should make decisions?

What are the criteria for decision making?

Who has access to databases?

With hospitals and health care agencies facing difficult ethical questions posed by the technological expansion, the U.S. Congress has studied the question of how the nation should develop, apply, and utilize the new technologies. Subcommittees of the House of Representatives have discussed the major questions such as who will decide how far technology should be developed, how the knowledge and technology should be used, and who should benefit from it.

More than 600 births worldwide via in-vitro fertilization have occurred since the technique was begun in 1978. About 2.5 million couples in the United States may be infertile and about forty percent of these could benefit from fertilization techniques according to leading scientists. However, treatment is expensive and the chance of becoming pregnant is low, less than 20%. Some politicians argue that funds should be available for such procedures.

Hospitals are encouraged to have active ethics committees to address ethical concerns. The committee should determine policies and monitor implementation of those policies. As medical technology and knowledge expand, these committees may also have to educate staff and clients about the ethical, medical, and legal issues surrounding such techniques as genetic engineering or therapy.

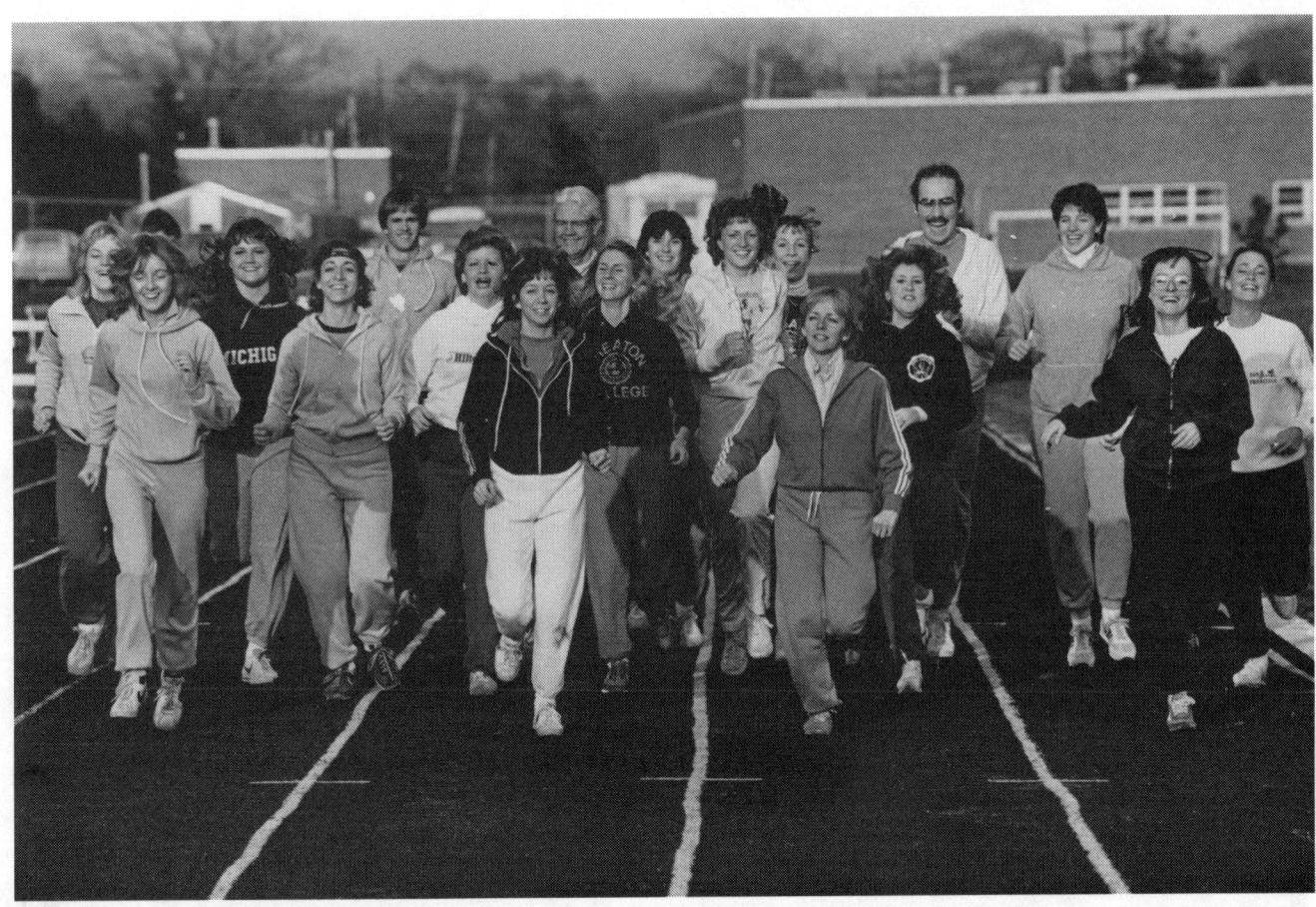

Who gets screened? And who decides?

Taking a Position on Eugenics

Each of the discussed perspectives is in itself complex. When persons of varying perspectives attempt to reach "consensus," a positive, a negative, or a middle-of-the-road approach to the use of eugenics may result. The pro-eugenics approach encourages the "fit" of a society to have many children in the effort to improve the human race.

Positive Eugenics Efforts

- incentives for educated women to bear children
- special admissions criteria to higher education for those persons deemed "fit"
- computer dating services
- asserting the relationship of IQ with heredity
- in-vitro fertilization
- artificial insemination
- freezing of gametes for future use
- prenatal diagnosis of genetic disease

The negative position proposes a variety of techniques to achieve the purpose of "preventing the unfit" from having children.

Negative Eugenics Techniques

- encouraging less-educated women to have smaller families
- sterilization, either voluntary or involuntary
- prenatal testing, which enables women to become aware of and abort a fetus that would be born with an inherited disability
- marriage restriction
- segregation through institutionalization
- euthanasia

The middle-of-the-road position suggests that eugenics techniques could be utilized under certain conditions, provided a model for decision making could be developed. Decision making should take into account the humanity of the patient, the heritability measure of human traits — the measure value can vary depending on the range of environments — and that the heritability of traits does not imply the immutability of a trait (Chan, 1985).

Alma and the Dating Service

An elite computer dating service advertises that it will match people for intellectual and physical considerations (height, musculature, and coloration). The ad specifies that people with limited mental facilities and/or physical difficulties should not apply. A sizable fee is charged, and a lengthy investigation is conducted. The service guarantees success.

Alma applies to this service. She is an "A" student, but since birth she has had a severe hearing problem. When this problem was detected during the investigation, Alma was rejected. She was told that her registration fee was nonrefundable because the company specified that people with limited mental facilities and/or physical difficulties should not apply.

What should Alma do? Does she have any rights?

Making Decisions about Eugenics

Decisions about eugenics must be made at various levels:

- at the personal level, as individuals
- at the social level, as groups (social and political entities or organizations)
- as a national body of people, as the United States
- at the global level, as a human species

In those deliberations the following questions need to be considered:

Are mental and physical diseases and social problems based on biological factors and inherited?

Some researchers argue that not all mental and physical disease are based in biological factors and are therefore not inherited. The assumption then that persons with these afflictions should be identified for intervention would need to be questioned. While social problems such as alcoholism or drug abuse may have some relationship to hereditary factors, it should not be assumed that all social problems have biological bases.

Could preoccupation with inherited diseases lead to increased disregard of societal threats (accidents at work, home, on the street, or lifestyle) which disable or kill persons routinely?

At times we seem to forget that we live in a society in which every day people of all ages become disabled or killed by accidents at home, at work, or on the streets and highways. Many of the accidents could have been prevented if the necessary money were spent and the necessary precautions taken. If society focuses on genetic-related problems and neglects disabilities which could be prevented, the possibility exists that more people disabled by accidents could have been aided than persons with genetic problems.

Is it in our interest to decide not just whether we bear a child, but what kind of child we bear?

The surrogate motherhood option to having babies has yielded some contracts wherein the father wants a perfect baby which has his genes. Stipulations that the contract mother will abort the fetus if there is evidence that the fetus is not up to standard have been written. No other category of father — natural, step or adoptive — can lay down such criteria. Do persons have a right to a perfect child or do they only have a right to try to have one?

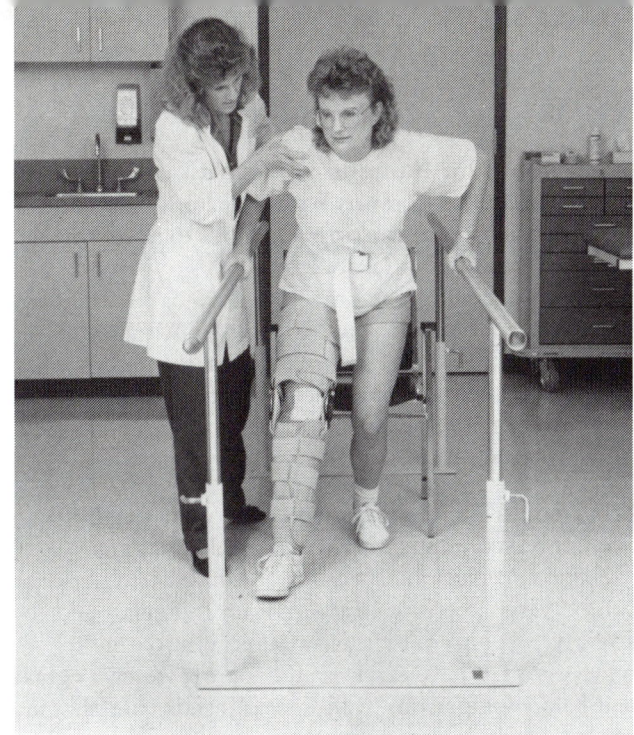

Accidents disable people every day.

Who should make the judgments regarding "fitness" or "unfitness"?

Scientists and physicians worldwide are developing technologies that could be used to decide which lives are worth living and who should or should not inhabit the world. They have provided the tools. Pregnant women have been making the choices up to now and for the most part have not been forced into the decisions. Should other persons — church leaders, politicians, scientists – be involved in the decision making?

Who has the right to determine who should and should not live in the global society?

The intertwining of the economic, political, and social systems of the nations of the world has led to an increased mixing of the philosophical, moral, and ethical systems as well. No longer can nations ignore global implications for their actions. Decision making has been expanded to include the global perspective. Therefore, decisions may have to be made for the global society as well.

What is the public's role in the decision-making process and in the enforcement of the decisions?

The American public has not been considered to be proactive in accepting responsibility for making decisions at the societal level. It has been easy to relinquish personal and public decision making to others and then to react to those decisions. Should greater emphasis be placed on discovering how society feels or thinks about genetic therapy, prior to decisions being made which likely would have effect upon individuals?

What should a humane society do to meet the requirements of persons with special needs and to provide them with the opportunities to accept their rights as members of a society?

For many of us, a great risk is that we or our children will acquire a disability during our lives. Would it be in the interest of all to have services exist for people with special needs and to respect their civil rights when they're seeking employment or participating in activities of the society?

What could happen when people with disabilities are perceived as social and economic burdens?

Services to meet the special needs of disabled persons can be very expensive to the individual families and to society. Technical innovations could make it unnecessary to have services and appropriate civil rights legislation for persons with special needs, but should society decide to support such innovations?

Do all persons want to know about their hereditary traits and what implications these have for their unborn children? Or would the majority of people prefer to be ignorant about eugenics?

A random, scientific sampling of 1464 adult Americans in 1986 found strong resistance to choosing the sex of babies, a choice now possible as a result of in-vitro fertilization techniques. Seventy-two percent said they would not take the opportunity to do so. Other surveys regarding genetic screening prior to birth indicated that most people would rather not know about themselves and their unborn children. Most parents would refuse abortion in the case of a normal fetus carrying a single copy of a mutant gene for phenylketonuria. The prospect of eliminating this genetic disease is slight, as a result.

The mutation responsible for Huntington's disease is quite rare. With more and better genetic probes and markers being identified, elective abortion of all affected fetuses in known families could lead to Huntington's disease being practically eliminated in a short period of time.

If specific areas of eugenics — genetic engineering, genetic-defect detection — were used altruistically only, could we as individuals and as a global community accept this concept?

If assurances could be obtained that the innovative technologies would only be used for "goodness" and for the benefit of persons, would it be easier for you to accept the use of the techniques?

What is the likelihood of losing sight of the individual while trying to improve humankind?

Textbooks in ethics have long used the moral principles that each person counts as one, and none counts for more or less than one. A typical example of the principle was the hypothetical case of a hospital with five patients, four of them persons of world-class accomplishments (a statesman, musician, mathematician, and philosopher), and the fifth, a mentally deficient person without kin or means. The fifth patient does, however, have healthy organs which, if transplanted, could save the lives of the other four. The point was that it would not be right to kill the one in order to save the other four, for people are always to be treated as entities and never as means.

It has been a revered principle in the history of the United States. Today, however, the principle is becoming an hypothesis.

What if one undesirable trait coexisted with other highly desirable characteristics?

Could we assign relative values to the specific traits?

Is there a need to examine judicial assumptions supporting decisions made in the 1930s and 1940s that are alien to our current values?

A number of legal questions need to be addressed in view of current social and personal value systems. For example, does the legal definition of "parents" reflect current or historic values? A definition of who can be the defendant if a baby is born that suffers mental or physical defects needs to be reviewed. What will be the legal status of spare embryos not used in the the in vitro fertilization procedures, who will own them, and who will decide how they are used or disposed of? Concerning sperm banks, who has the rights and what rights should be considered in deciding how the sperm can be used?

The rights of surrogate or "host" mothers as well as the legal status of the resultant child need to be determined. While some legal distinctions between legitimate and illegitimate children have been removed, many remain and in some parts of society a social stigma may attach to an illegitimate child and/or its parents.

Differences between the values inherent in existing laws and regulations and the current values should be reviewed. Problems can exist when principles of fundamental law are founded only on unanchored reason or sentiment.

Is it appropriate for decisions that influence the lives of the collective body of humanity to be made behind closed doors by professions, research review panels, or funding agencies?

Major universities have committees to monitor faculty research. Health care organizations have committees that review their members. State and Federal governments have agencies that regulate certain research activities. Agencies that fund research frequently have panels to review proposals and projects. However, most decisions of these groups are the result of meetings which are not attended by the public. Indeed the public may not be aware of the existence of such groups or their decisions until long after the fact. Should the public have more access to the decision-making process of such groups?

What role does individual freedom or sovereignty play in research?

The laboratories of the researchers and scientists have long been viewed as private domain. The freedom to explore, develop, and create has been acknowledged and supported. However, the explosion of new technologies has led to questions regarding the ethical considerations for the application of such knowledge.

What are the potential misuses/abuses of research findings/products?

"And so . . . we are facing questions for which we have no ready answers. The questions are being answered, however. Most of us, probably because we want to live with a clear conscience, prefer not to think about the answers that are being given. Later, we can say that we did not know."

Neuhaus. 1988, p. 26

Should human hereditary traits be enhanced? There is no hard-and-fast answer. Nevertheless, three suggestions for personal and social/political decision making are offered here:

1. Gain awareness of the potentialities and consequences of the technologies and knowledges.

2. If in doubt, go slowly in the applications of the knowledges and technological processes.

3. Recognize that the democratic government in America is based on *four branches* of power: legislative, judicial, administrative, and the citizenry. The first three elements are responsible to the last one. Ultimately, the citizenry, as individuals and members of national and global communities, must make the decision regarding the issues and questions related to eugenics.

Summary

Eugenics, the study of hereditary improvement emerged in the late nineteenth century and gained its greatest influence in the United States in the early 1900s. With the primary aim of the "betterment" of the human race, the eugenics movement has become a focus of attention once again in the 1980s.

The multiple factors involved with the issue include such perspectives as political/legal, economic, social, scientific, and philosophical/moral/ethical. These elements have impact and implications for decision making at various levels, e.g., personal, social, and political.

Technological advances have led to increasing concern for the moral, legal, and ethical issues involved in the application of the technologies for the betterment of the human race. Researchers, persons in government, theologians, lawyers, and others are expressing a need for enhancing the awareness of consequences of advanced technology applications.

Our democratic government is based upon four components or branches: administrative, judicial, legislative, and the citizenry. The first three branches are responsible to the latter one. Ultimately, the citizenry, as individuals and a collective body, must make the decisions on questions and issues related to eugenics and the implications for the individual and society.

Cited References

Chan, C. (1985). Eugenics on the rise: a report from Singapore. *International Journal of Health Services,* 15(4): 707-12.

Chomsky, (Ed.), (1983, June). The unborn generations — humanity or convenience? *Nursing Mirror,* 156(22):23-29.

Hubbard, R. (1986). Eugenics and prenatal testing. *International Journal of Health Services,* 16(2): 227-42.

Huxley, J. (1941). The vital importance of eugenics. *Harper's Monthly,* 163:324-31.

Melendy, M. (1904). *The science of eugenics and sex life.* Unknown: Vansant.

Merz, B. (1984, October 8). Gene therapy: correcting the errors in life's blue print. *Medical World News,* 125(19): 46-62.

Neuhaus, R. (1988, April). The return of eugenics. *Commentary,* 85: 15-26.

Talbot, L. (1983, January). Boy or girl — is it possible to choose? *Nursing Mirror,* 156 (3): 32-36.

Terman, L. (1924). The conservation of talent. *School and Society,* 29 (483): 363. Cited on p. 108 of S. Rose. Scientific racism and ideology: the IQ racket from Galton to Jensen. In *Ideology of/in the natural sciences,* 87-116. Cambridge, Mass.: Schenkman, 1980.

Wallace, D. (1984, October). Congress examines ethical issues given birth by genetic engineering. *Modern Healthcare,* 14(13): 114-15.

Additional Bibliography

Applegate, M., and Entrekin, N. (1984). Case studies for students: a companion to teaching ethics in nursing. *National League of Nursing,* 41: 1963A, 1-36.

Becker, W. (Producer), (1975). *Genetic engineering: the research that shouldn't be done?* Indianapolis, Indiana Committee for the Humanities.

Berry, A., and Peter, J. (1984, March). DNA probes for infectious disease. *Diagnostic Medicine,* 7 (3): 62-66, 68, 70-72.

Breathnach, C. (1985). Biographical sketches — 55: Galton. *Irish Medical Journal,* 78 (8): 238.

Clark, M., and Doi, A. (1983, May 30). Choosing your child's sex. *Newsweek,* 101 (22): 102.

Cook, R. (1986, November 16). Gene therapy — hope for the hopeless? *The Indianapolis Star,* 18A.

Cuisine, D. (1982). Legal Implications, in *Developments in Human Reproduction and their Eugenic, Ethical Implications,* Carter, C. (Ed.), Academic Press, New York.

Cynkar, R. (1981). Buck v. Bell: "felt necessities" v. fundamental values. *Columbia Law Review,* 81: 1418-61.

DeYoung, H. (1986, August). In search of a winning strategy. *High Technology,* 45-46.

Gene-splicing techniques cure the shivers in mice. (1987, March 11). *The Chronicle of Higher Education,* 23:28, 7.

Genes responsible for retinal cancer and muscular dystrophy are located. (1986, October 22). *The Chronicle of Higher Education,* 23:8, 5.

Heaney, R., and Barger-Lux, M. (1984, Fall). Today's crisis in university-provided education in the health professions. *Educational Record,* 42-47.

Holzman, D. (1986, November 17). Grafting cures to genetic diseases. *Insight,* 58-59.

Holzman, D. (1987, November 9). Prenatal tests carry hard choices. *Insight.* 51-52.

Indiana Committee for the Humanities (Producer). *Controlling heredity: genetic research and its implications for the individual and society.* Indianapolis, 1976.

Karp, L. (1982, June). Past perfect. *American Journal of Medical Genetics,* 12(2): 127-30.

Kotulak, R. (1986, October 3). DNA's long hidden secrets will herald revolution. *The Indianapolis Star,* 14.

Morris, W. (Ed.), (1980). *The American Heritage Dictionary of the English Language.* Boston: Mifflin.

Most Americans would refuse to pick baby's sex. (1986, November 18). *Tampa Tribune,* 1.

Namenwirth, M. (Producer), (1975). *Reproduction in the 21st century.* Indianapolis: Indiana Committee for the Humanities.

Pope says scientists can't ignore moral and ethical considerations. (1987, May). *Indianapolis Star,* 1.

Predetermining a baby's gender. (1986, September). *Parade.*

Reilly, P. (1983, Summer). The surgical solution: the writings of the activist physicians in the early days of eugenical sterilization. *Perspectives in Biology and Medicine,* 26(4): 637-56.

Reilly, P. (1983, December). The Virginia Racial Integrity Act revisited. *American Journal of Medical Genetics, 16* (4): 483-92.

Robertson, M. (1984, February 11). Towards a medical eugenics. *British Medical Journal,* 288 (6415): 429-30.

Too Many Children. (1987, June 1). *Insight,* 39.

Valenza, C. (1985, January-February). Was Margaret Sanger a racist? *Family Planning Perspective,* 17(1): 44-46.

Vatican document on birth technology unlikely to alter research, ethicists say. (1987, March), *The Chronicle of Higher Education,* 6.

Wheeler, D. (1986, September 3). Researchers weigh a stepped-up effort to map the terrain of the human gene. *The Chronicle of Higher Education,* 32-34.

The Dictator and the Boys

A *Third World country has a lengthy civil war in which many young men are killed. Once the war is over, the dictator in power decides to address the problem of the low number of males in his country. He decrees that the people should have only male babies. He also wants only healthy babies so he specifies that prospective parents will have to be checked to ensure that they are in good health. Until they are approved by the doctors, they cannot be parents. If a prospective father does not pass the physical and mental requirements, sperm will be supplied from a sperm bank. If the mother does not pass, she will have a test tube baby implanted. The sperm may be her husband's or not depending on whether he passes the state's requirements. If someone becomes pregnant without being evaluated, the fetus will be aborted. In addition, the police will enforce the decree by giving a warning after the first offense and a jail sentence the second time.*

The dictator arranges to have a major world power provide the medical expertise needed to put this program into operation. In exchange for that power's assistance, he agrees to allow that country to mine the minerals in his country for a specified period.

- Who should establish the criteria for the male donors?

- What should be the standards for the male and female biological parents?

- Would the parents love a child whose parentage was unknown as much as they would their own biological child?

- What effect would such a program have on a family structure?

- Does a country have the right to decree the gender of a child?

- Should the rest of the world stand by and watch this type of child production?

- What moral and ethical responsibilities do world powers have?

- Is there such a thing as universal human rights?

- Could this situation ever occur in the United States?

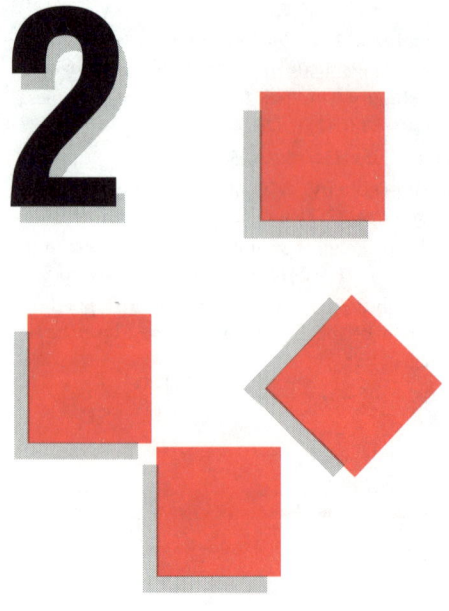

Splicing Genes to Understand, Interpret, and Change Nature

Paul D. Hoeksema*

Objectives

After reading this chapter, you should be able to:

- Define the terms listed at the beginning of this chapter.

- List three bioengineered products that are currently in use to correct life-threatening human physical conditions.

- Describe why scientists would want to change the genetic makeup of certain cells in the human body.

- Discuss two concerns that illustrate the need for protective steps when scientists use recombinant DNA technology.

- Formulate a statement to guide scientists in determining which changes in organisms are appropriate to initiate.

Terms and Definitions

Amino acid. One of many biochemicals that are building blocks for proteins.
Antibody. A substance made in an organism to neutralize toxins, bacteria, and other foreign entities.
Applied scientist. A person who develops practical uses for specific scientific information.
Bioengineer. A scientist who splices genetic material to develop a useful drug, cure a hereditary disease, or change some life form.
DNA. Stands for deoxyribonucleic acid, the component of genes that controls heredity.
Gene. The part of a chromosome that transmits hereditary traits.
Gene splicing. Replacement of DNA sections of a gene to introduce a different genetic expression.
Immune response. Use of antibodies already present or injected to neutralize or destroy disease-causing materials.
Interferon. Specific antibody injected to neutralize or destroy disease-causing materials.
Monoclone. Host units with reformatted DNA coded to produce a drug or other chemical product.

Recombinant DNA. Restructured genetic material formed when new DNA sections are spliced into existing strands.

Research scientist. A person who conducts experiments, adding to available scientific information, without necessarily recognizing an immediate use for the results.

Restriction enzyme. A digesting substance that assists in separating DNA sections so new strands can be reconstructed.

*Paul D. Hoeksema
Allied Health Teacher Educator, Ferris State University, Big Rapids, MI 49307.

Introduction

Scientists who work in laboratories to change the genetic makeup of organisms are called **gene-splicers**. This **bioengineering process** is being used to produce such biochemicals as human growth hormone, insulin, and other vaccines and drugs to treat human diseases. It could ultimately be used to change a genetic arrangement, prevent or correct a condition or disease by deleting the effect, or provide new genetic material to replace the genes that cause the trouble. Since small organisms like bacteria and viruses may be used to carry the new genetic material, there is concern that changes intended for one organism could affect others or be released into the environment. This might result in undesirable changes that would cause more trouble than they correct. Identity tags are now used to track recombinant DNA in the environment to provide a measure of genetic safety. When the potential changes alter human genetic characteristics, even more concern is raised. Bioengineers should be fully aware of the outcome of their experiments and then use the technology and its products wisely.

Recombinant DNA Technology: An Overview

The principal ingredient of heredity-bearing **genes** is the **DNA molecule**. This molecule can be compared to a ladder in which the sequential arrangement of rungs and sides determines a genetic code controlling what each cell will be and do (see accompanying figure). Research has accomplished the purification of **restriction enzymes**. These enzymes act as chemical knives and cut the delicate DNA at specific positions into neat pieces with very sticky ends. Mixing pieces of DNA from different organisms and regluing them by **DNA ligase** result in the construction of tiny new genetic packages known as **recombinant DNA:** hence the process if referred to as **recombinant DNA technology**. The organism that ends up with this DNA in its cells will be and do what the reconstructed code directs.

Recombinant DNA technology is one of the biotechnologies that uses living organisms to carry out chemical processes or produce useful substances. **Bioprocess technology** has been around for many years; bread, cheese, and alcohol are recognized among its useful products. **Monoclonal antibody technology** informs scientists how to fuse cancer cells with cells that produce a particular antibody. These fused cells proliferate and, in a short time, produce the particular antibody in large quantities. It is hoped the antibodies will be present in sufficient quantity to destroy specific cancer cells without harming normal cells and tissues.

Recombinant DNA technology transfers specific pieces of DNA coding for a particular protein into a host organism. Before a transfer can be accomplished, the genes that code for the desired proteins must be identified. Scientists frequently identify the amino acid sequence of the protein ultimately desired and then work backward to the nucleotide sequence to identify the gene to be transferred.

Once the genes are identified, they must be isolated. Restriction enzymes recognize and cut very specific DNA sequences out of DNA strands. These sequences can later be moved into host organisms. The **plasmid**, a ring-shaped piece of DNA found naturally in most bacteria, is most frequently used to accomplish this transfer. The plasmids are cut using the same enzymes used to clip out the selected gene. The sticky ends of

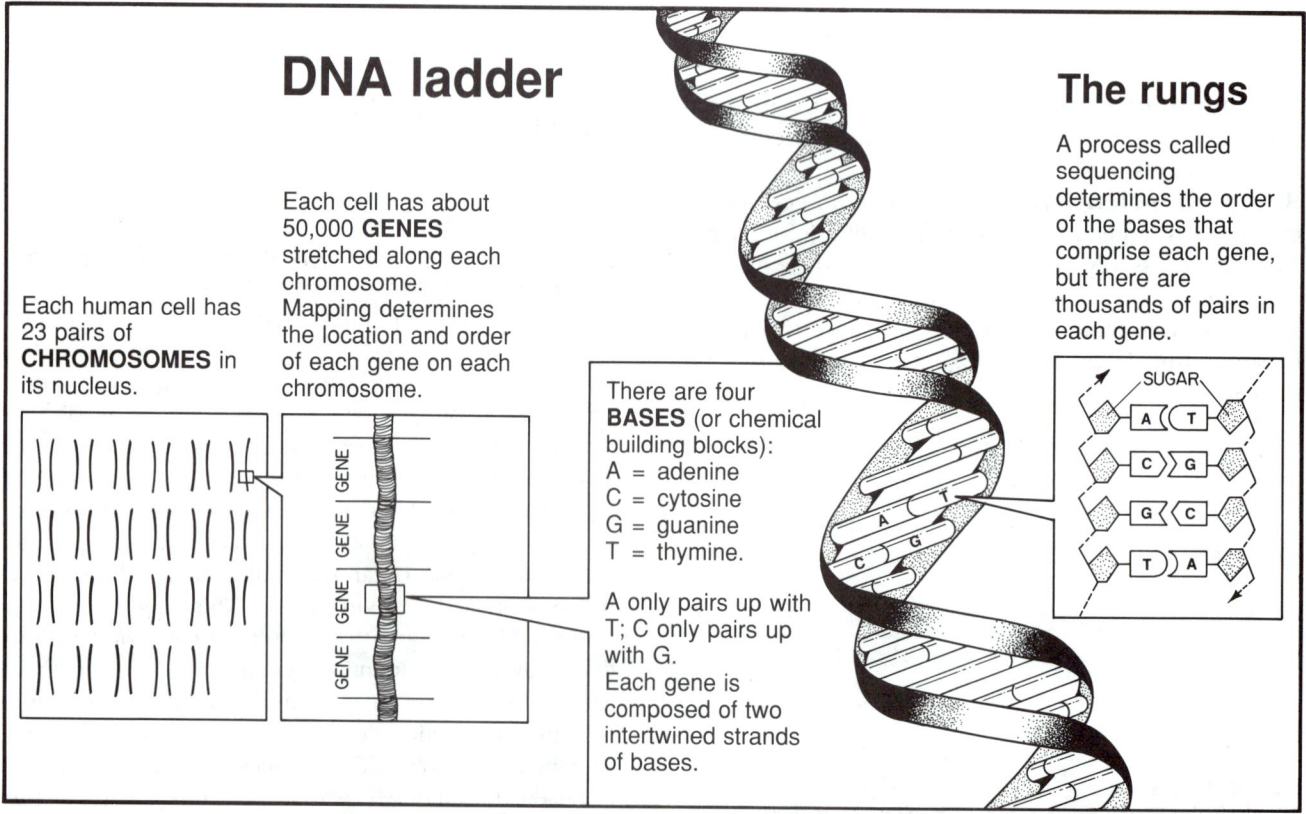

The ability to identify rungs (or base pairs) of the DNA ladder has led to significant and rapid breakthroughs in understanding genetics.

the plasmid match the sticky ends of the gene. When the cut plasmid and genes are mixed together, it is possible for these pieces to be brought together, their complementary base pairs joined by **hydrogen bonding.** When the appropriate bond has been formed and the new code has been incorporated, the plasmid is mixed with a host organism. There the plasmids are replicated, the gene becomes active, and the host now produces the protein coded by the inserted gene.

Rapid multiplication of the altered host microorganisms under laboratory conditions can result in the harvesting of unlimited quantities of desired cell products. This process not only allows the production of test tube antibodies, but also the possibility of eventually synthesizing the very genes that are determinants of hereditary features.

yet another enzyme defect. To take a hypothetical example of the disastrous effects of an error originating in the laboratory: What would happen if a genetic recombination produced a deadly poison in *E. coli,* the poison was allowed to multiply, and the hybrid found its way into a sewer system where unaltered *E. coli* also thrives?

Complete understanding of many defects will undoubtedly lead to the correction of inherited human conditions before they are manifested in the individual. It can also result in the synthesis or copying of a gene for production in or transfer through a bacterium or for direct insertion into humans.

Altered Gene Expression in *E. coli*

The bacteria **E. coli** has frequently been used as a host cell for the desired expressions of foreign genes. More is known about the control of gene expression in this organism than in any other, and it easily exchanges genetic material with other bacteria. It just so happens that *E. coli* is common in the digestive system of humans and is also found in every other warm-blooded animal, in insects, and in fish. There was certainly a need to develop a seriously weakened mutant strain of *E. coli* for use in recombinant DNA experiments. That strain would need to self-destruct outside the laboratory to reduce the chances of deadly material being released in the world through poor laboratory technique. The versatility of *E. coli* is illustrated in the account of the laboratory processes used to develop "safe" organisms (see box).

Despite the studies made with *E. coli* the search for better — or more defective — microbes continues.

A single error in the genetic code, a part improperly sequenced or misplaced by nature or in the laboratory, can induce a complicated disease involving several organs. It can lead to the production of the wrong kind of protein or a flawed one. In **Down's syndrome** more genes than nature intended may be present, and in multiple inherited defects some genes may be missing. In **phenylketonuria (PKU)** an enzyme defect results in an inability to convert an amino acid into another material. The amino acid collects, breaks down, and interferes with normal brain development. In **galactosemia** sugar cannot be properly used owing to

---

The Challenges of Developing a Safe Strain of E. coli

First an *E. coli* with a gene deficiency preventing it from making **diaminopimelic acid (DAP)**, an important ingredient of the protective membrane, was developed. Without DAP, the organisms swell and burst during normal growth.

Unfortunately, some of the mutants, descendants of the new microbe, mutated naturally and began making their own DAP. Through the deletion of another gene, a strain resulted that remained DAPless.

However, these mutants survived and reproduced without DAP. They made a sticky substance called **colanic acid** which held them together in the absence of a normal outer membrane.

By manipulating another gene, the microbe was rendered incapable of making colanic acid with an unexpected dividend — extreme sensitivity to ultraviolet light. Finally, what seemed to be a safe research bacteria was produced.

However, even dying *E. coli* can conjugate with healthy ones, transferring potentially dangerous genetic material in the process. When the capacity to make thymine was deleted, genes could not be passed to healthy outsiders. These tailor-made bacteria cannot live outside the laboratory, and are not able to colonize or even live in the human intestinal tract. They cannot survive in human serum and are destroyed by common household detergents.

Is It Safe? Is It Ethical?

There is a distinct difference between reprogramming a bacterium to make biochemicals and redesigning the human race through utilization of recombinant DNA techniques. In the scientific community, the most persistent concern has been for public safety. Most bacterial change through genetic reconstruction has been no more exotic than what typically occurs in nature. The chances of producing viable new organisms accidentally by gene splicing seems negligible, but gene splicing and gene therapy inevitably carry the risk of a forbidden play without recognizing what the forfeit will be. Much more to be feared are the possibilities of deliberate misuse and abuse.

Although gene copying will certainly wipe out many inherited diseases in the future, it could also be used more insidiously for intentionally lowering human intelligence. Scientists have lined up on both sides of the ethical issues. Temporary bans have halted potentially dangerous and not so dangerous experiments, as research is evaluated under safety guidelines and regulations are supervised by the Environmental Protection Agency, the Department of Agriculture, and the Food and Drug Administration. The emerging genetic biotechnology industry is one of the most heavily regulated in the United States.

Applications of Recombinant DNA Products

Recombinant DNA is currently being used to produce drugs and vaccines, some approved for human use, and a laboratory animal:

- Production of **human growth hormone (hGH)** in *E. coli* which is at least as active as authentic hGH for the treatment of dwarfism due to growth hormone deficiency. The hGH had previously been available only from cadavers.

- On October 29, 1980, the Food and Drug Administration approved marketing **Humulin**, the only animal protein made in a bacteria in such a way that its structure is identical to that of the natural insulin molecule. Up to the time of the development of the recombinant DNA technique, insulin has only been available from animal pancreases.

- On July 23, 1986, the Food and Drug Administration approved a **genetically engineered vaccine to prevent hepatitis B.** This product is the first engineered vaccine from a source other than blood plasma approved for human use. Its use removes

---

The Lottery and Genetics

Jim and Joan win the lottery. Jim quits his job as a bus driver. Joan calls the restaurant where she works as a waitress and tells her boss exactly what she thinks of him and that she will not be working there anymore.

The couple decides to travel. While in a foreign country, they read about a scientist who is conducting experiments in genetic engineering. This doctor maintains that, for a price, he can guarantee the sex, intelligence, general physical characteristics, and talents of a baby.

Having no children and thinking they would like to start a family, Joan and Jim are considering this approach as a way of ensuring that they get exactly what they want in a baby.

What are some of the points they should consider in deciding whether or not to use the services of the doctor?

lingering fears of catching other conditions such as AIDS from a hepatitis innoculant derived from human blood plasma.

- **Tissue plasminogen activator (TPA),** a bioengineered substance, has been given experimentally to dissolve blood clots and renew critical blood flow to reduce tissue destruction in heart attack victims. TPA is marketed under the name **Activase.** Its cost is ten times that of **streptokinase,** a treatment competitor not made by genetic engineering. Although one dose of TPA is reported to cost $2,200, only one treatment is needed. First evidence has been presented to confirm that the drug significantly reduces deaths following heart attacks.

- On November 11, 1986, a television news report indicated that scientists in Argentina had injected cows with a **DNA-engineered rabies vaccine**. In April, 1986, the United States Department of Agriculture had halted sale of **Omnivac PRV,** a new genetically engineered viral vaccine being used to immunize swine against pseudorabies.

- In April 1988, the U.S. Patent Office assigned the first patent on a **laboratory mouse, created by recombinant DNA technology.** This mouse is more susceptible to agents causing breast cancer than other mice are and will be extremely useful in analyzing the relationships between environmental and hereditary causes of cancer. Conclusions to these studies may result in improved diagnostic tools for human cancer. Twenty-one other patent applications are now pending for new bioengineered animals.

By July 1988, nine drugs and vaccines had been approved for human use by the Food and Drug Administration. These products and the health problem treated are:

- Monoclate — hemophilia
- Humulin — diabetes
- Humatrope — human growth hormone deficiency in children
- Protropin — human growth hormone deficiency in children

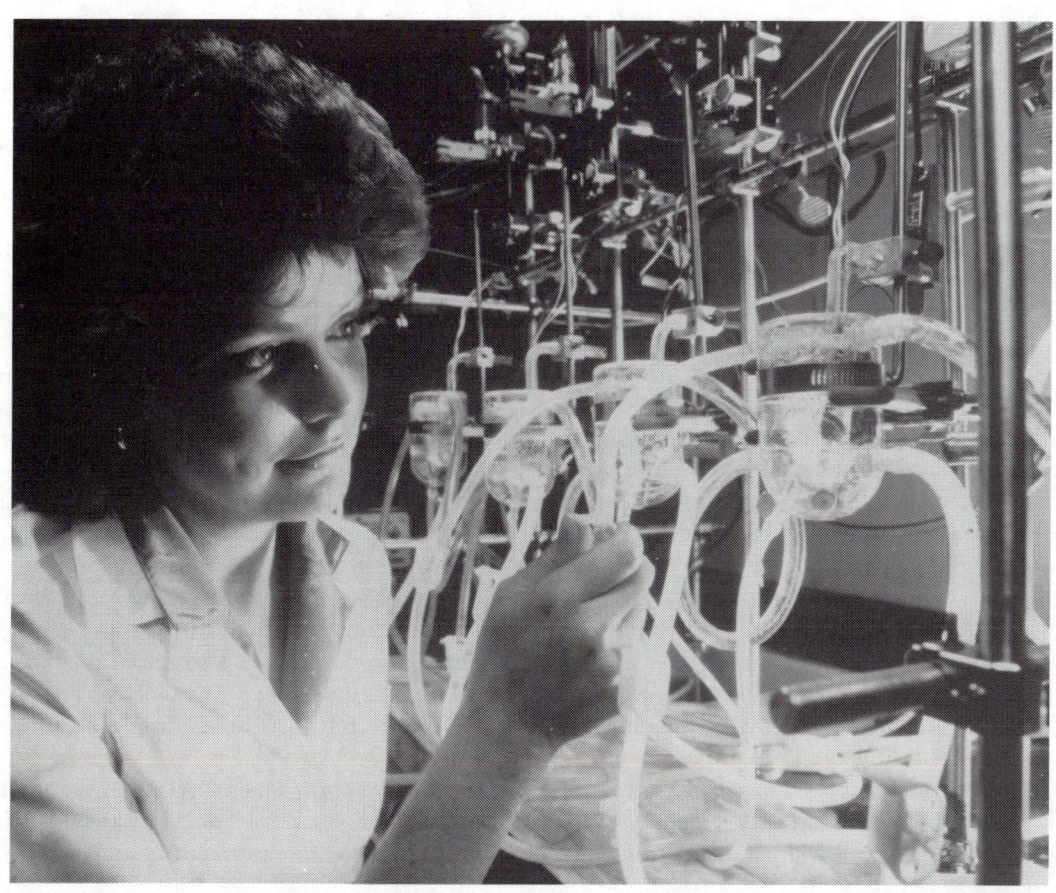

- Activase — acute myocardial infarction
- Roferon-A — hairy cell leukemia
- Recombivax HB — hepatitis B vaccine
- Orthoclone OKT3 — kidney transplant rejection
- Intron-A — hairy cell leukemia and chronic myelogenous leukemia

At least eighty-one other products are in the final stages of development — all products of bioengineering technology.

Another promising development is the application of recombinant DNA technology to the treatment of cancer. By producing **monoclonal antibodies**, antibodies with reformatted DNA, and injecting them into individuals as **interferons**, it is possible to improve immune function and attack tumors. Clinical use of interferons has been limited because of the difficulty in obtaining the material for target diseases. Interferon has also proved useful in suppressing the migration of **leukocytes** (white blood cells) and for its general antiviral and antiproliferative effects.

The human immune system, unlike other systems, cannot be characterized as a defined anatomic entity within which specific physiologic functions are contained or effected. The system's one trillion lymphocytes of varied subsets, secretory products, and regulatory chemical substances are all responsible for specific immune functions. These cells move freely in and out of the blood and lymphoid channels, giving the immune system the capability of carrying out its functions for health within all body tissues.

The use of **interleukin-2 (IL-2)** in a controversial immunotherapy has resulted in striking improvements in some patients with advanced cases of cancer. The IL-2 is a naturally produced substance "manufactured" by genetic engineering techniques. The treatments bolster the immune system, which has already produced small amounts of IL-2. When white cells, the principal agents of the immune system, are separated from withdrawn blood and bathed in IL-2, they reproduce faster. Now known as lymphokine-activated killer cells, they are attracted to cancer cells and promptly destroy them. With controlled dosages, the toxic side effects of IL-2 can be controlled. FDA approval is needed to treat those patients who have metastatic kidney cancer and melanoma, conditions which appear to be most susceptible to the treatments.

The use of human interferons may ultimately provide a solution for **AIDS** treatment. The AIDS virus mutates frequently, changing the structure of its surface antigens so rapidly that the immune system cannot alter its antibodies fast enough to keep up with the disease. Its ability to move from cell to cell without first returning to the blood also makes the virus difficult to intercept. In the cell it is presently safe from antibodies produced to destroy it and from splicing to turn the immune system back on. As scientists improve their techniques they may be able to solve these puzzles.

The Use of Gene Therapy

DNA is the chemical material that controls a vast array of genetic information — from the type of metabolic enzymes that will be present in our bodies to the color of our eyes, hair, and skin. Sometimes the genetic coding goes awry, resulting in such abnormalities as defective, missing, or translocated genes. A **translocated gene** is one that is in the wrong position on the chromosome. Now in its infancy, the exciting field of **gene therapy** may one day permit scientists to correct such architectural errors of nature by inducing changes in the master blueprints of the body — the chromosomes.

In a hypothetical scenario, the therapy is used on an infant lacking the ADA gene, which is related to proper functioning of the immune system. The baby is put under general anesthesia and has up to 10 percent of its bone marrow removed (see accompanying diagram). The marrow is spun in a specially equipped centrifuge to isolate cells that scientists will try to repair with a modified virus. That virus has been altered to carry the missing gene. It contains enough viral machinery to "infect" the gene but contains none of the other virus qualities. After the bone marrow cells and altered viral particles have been combined in a petri dish and left for approximately twenty-four hours, the bone marrow cells with the new viral material are returned intravenously to the child's body. Blood tests will detect the presence of the enzyme specified by the new genetic material, transferred earlier, if the "infection" is successful.

Growing evidence suggests that in the future **gene therapy** will permit the treatment of severe and often fatal diseases through alteration of the DNA molecules that make up the genes and chromosomes. The list of human disorders that can be traced to a specific gene or gene region grows on a weekly basis.

A gene that produces a major component of **amyloid**, an abnormal protein, seems to be involved when the symptoms of **Alzheimer's disease** are present. This gene and recently identified markers for inherited Alzheimer's disease are located in the same

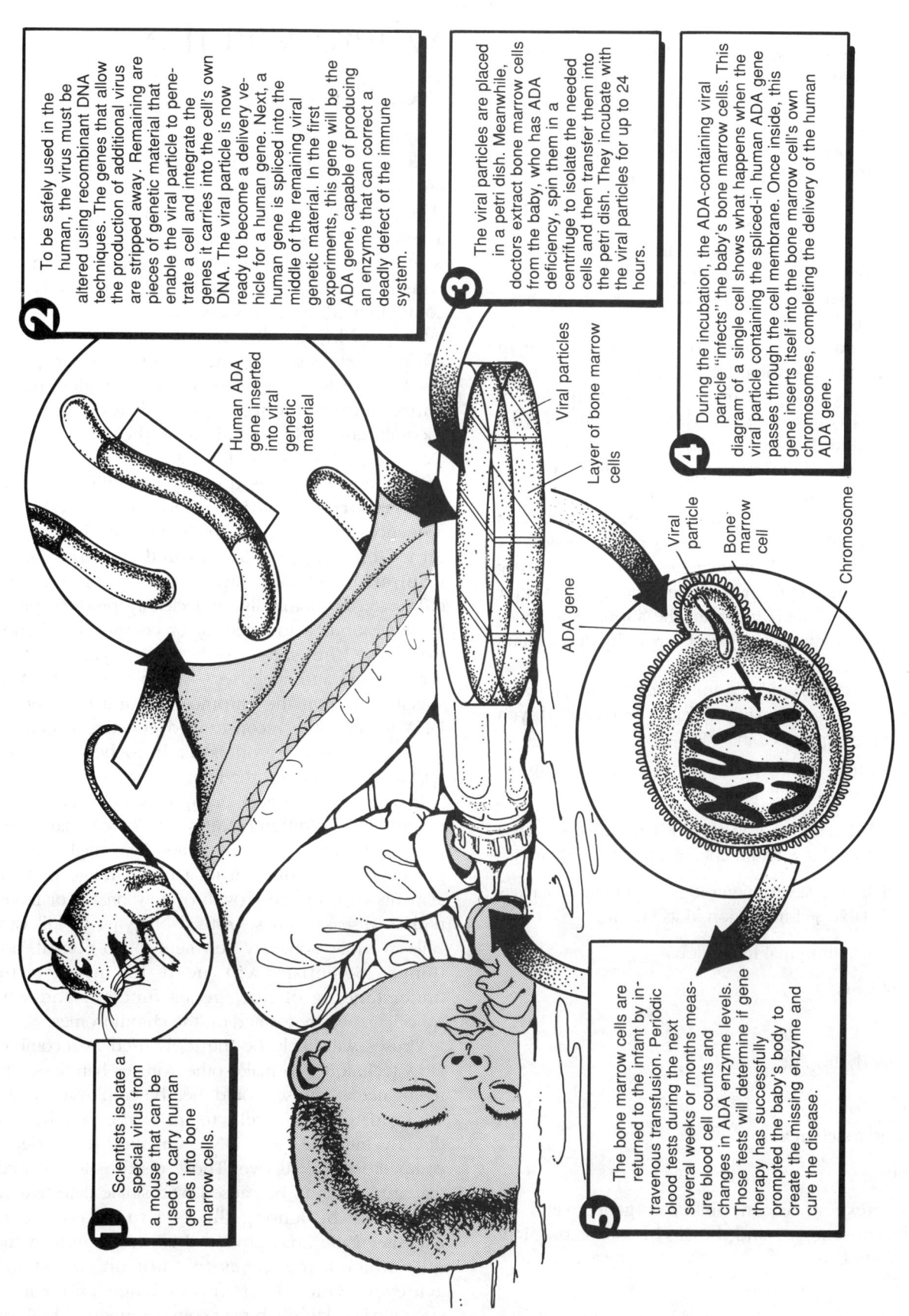

Gene therapy. Genetically reprogrammed viruses may someday be used by scientists to repair such defects as missing genes. (Reprinted with permission from the Washington Post.)

27

area of chromosome 21. Is the amyloid a by-product or a cause of the disease's ravages? There appear to be similarities between the symptoms in Alzheimer's and **Down's syndrome.** In each there is a unique tangled web of nerve cells in the brain, and Alzheimer's-like illness does occur in some patients having Down's syndrome. Whereas Down's syndrome is caused by the presence of an extra chromosome 21 or a translocated piece of the chromosome, it has been reported that Alzheimer's patients do not have more than the usual two copies of chromosome 21 or its parts. At one time it was thought that Down's and Alzheimer's might have the same cause.

The approximate location of a defective gene in humans that is responsible for a rare, inherited, cancer-causing disease and that may be a culprit in kidney cancer has been identified. This gene causes **Von Hippel Lundau disease.** People who have this disease develop cancers of different organs, including the brain and kidney. The finding promises to advance understanding of tumor-suppressing genes as protectors against cancer. If scientists are correct in their belief that the disease prevents certain genes involved in early organ development from becoming deactivated after they have served their function, the suppressor genes should serve as guardians against cancer by deactivating the defective genes.

Conditions that have been traced to specific genes or gene regions and that may ultimately be corrected with a gene therapy approach include:

- sickle-cell anemia, a blood disease causing an abnormality in the hemoglobin
- Tay-Sachs, a disorder of lipid metabolism that produces blindness and mental retardation early in life
- Lesch-Nyhan, a severe neurological illness that causes uncontrollable self-mutilation in its victim
- thalassemia, abnormal hemoglobin
- cystic fibrosis
- hemophilia
- muscular dystrophy
- cleft palate
- Huntington's chorea
- diabetes

Manic depression, recently linked to genetic sites on both chromosome 11 and the X chromosome, might also be treated.

Where Will the Research Lead?

The recombinant DNA technique is a means of interrupting nature, as well as interpreting it, of changing the world as well as attempting to understand it. Since 1973 the technique has advanced to a point where the ultimate potential effects are far more consequential than could have originally been contemplated. The process involves penetrating the nucleus of living cells, transplanting and rearranging nuclear acids, selecting and reinforcing desirable (and undesirable for that matter) characteristics from the entire natural genetic pool. Undoubtedly, the recombinant DNA technique is the most important technology of the twentieth century.

DNA engineering is used by two different groups. **The research scientist** expects to alter DNA gene sequences to learn how genes function, how they are turned off and on. **The applied scientist** plans to manipulate, change, and transfer genes to more efficiently, economically, and cleanly produce proteins by gene cloning for medical or commercial purposes. Both use the same tools — enzymes, ligases, polymerases, and nucleases — to split off the DNA from specific sites on the chromosome and to insert new DNA to form the reconstructed genetic material. The most immediate payoff is likely to be in medically related areas such as drug manufacture.

In the future, gene therapy may be applied to the control of cell differentiation and/or cellular activity, processes coded for by the genes. This might allow the prevention or correction of a broad range of human ailments — even the growth of new organs or limbs to replace diseased ones. Instead of trying to kill cancer cells, we may someday get them to do normal, useful things. Scientists will need to increase their understanding of how genes function and where specific genes are located on the chromosomes.

Viruses will likely be the tools used in recombinant DNA techniques to make other viruses harmless. These re-engineered viruses could then be employed to invade appropriate human cells to insert the healthy genes directly into the cell's DNA, enabling it to edge out competitors and survive. Those diseases and disorders that are known to be caused by a single defective gene will likely be among the first to be engineered. Experimentation has produced efficient transfer viruses, but inducing the genes to "turn on" is yet to be achieved. One never knows when and where a scientific breakthrough may come. Support of both basic research and clinical science can make these plausible options possible.

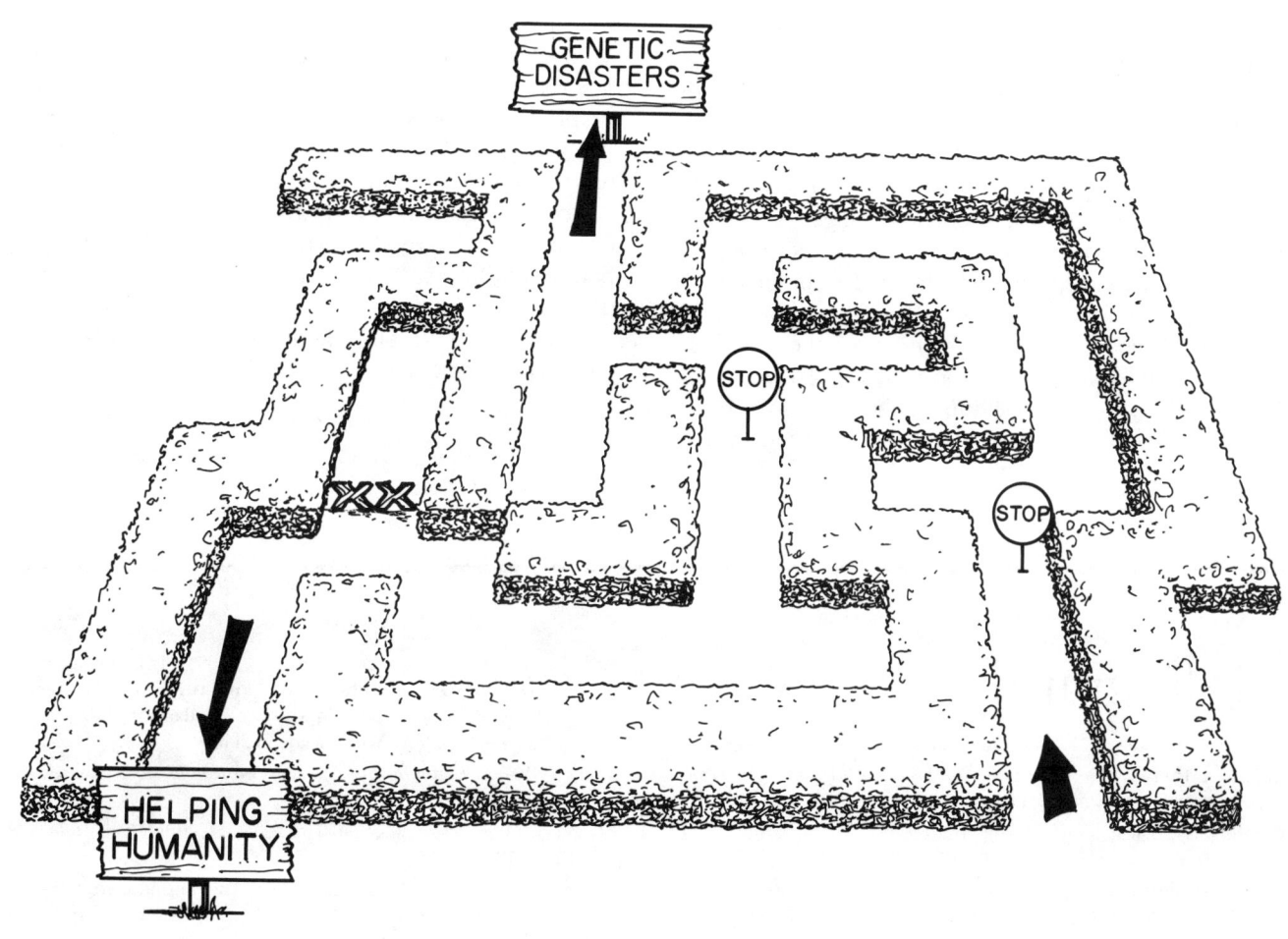

Summary

Recombinant DNA technology has resulted in the production of many bioengineered substances to replace drugs and vaccines, which have been costly and scarce or less desirable in treating many human conditions and diseases. The possibility of using bioengineered substances for effective treatment of such diseases as cancer and AIDS is particularly encouraging. The use to which present scientific findings are put will determine the ultimate value of this technology. Uncontrolled gene splicing which could result in ethical dilemmas will continue to be of scientific and societal concern. These concerns arise because the potential bioengineered changes alter the genetics of the human body itself and the condition of the environment in which we live. Questions that will need to be answered include:

Do scientists have the right to irreversibly change nature in order to satisfy individual curiosity and ambitions?

Who will determine which bioengineered products are useful and for what purpose?

Should scientists create novel life forms and then have the right to make, use, or sell the invention as a proprietary commodity?

Scientists who are genetic researchers are among the first to recognize opportunities for abuse.

Modified trait expressions and changed life forms may be expected to carry the recombined DNA into the gene pool of the future. What is accomplished today must be done wisely and carefully so that whatever happens in the future is predictable and achieved under ethically controlled conditions.

Bibliography

Baily, R. (1988, June 27). Ministry of fear. *Forbes,* 141 (14): 138-39.

Bollon, A. P. (1984). *Recombinant DNA products: insulin, interferon, and growth hormone.* Boca Raton, FL: CRC Press.

Carolina Biological Supply Company. (1985). *An introduction to genetic engineering — a teacher's manual.* Burlington, NC: Carolina Biological Supply Company.

Goodfield, J. (1977). *Playing God.* New York: Random House.

Gorman, C. (1988, April 25). A mouse that roared. *Time,* 131 (17): 83.

Hall, S. S. (1987, August). One potato patch that is making genetic history. *Smithsonian, (18(5): 125-36.*

Hapgood, F. (1887, November). Viruses emerge as new key for unlocking life's mysteries. *Smithsonian, 18 (8): 116-27.*

Howard, T., and Rifkin, J. (1977). *Who should play God?* New York: Delacorte Press.

Jaroff, L. (1986, April 21). Fighting the biotech wars. *Time,* 127 (16): 52-54.

Jaroff, L. (1989, March 20). The Gene Hunt. *Time.* 133 (12): 62-67.

Jenkins, C. L. (1987, April). Recombinant paper plasmids. *The Science Teacher,* 54 (4): 44-48.

Langone, J. (1978). *Human engineering, marvel or menace.* Boston: Little Brown.

Lathe, R. F., Lecocq, J. P., and Everett, R. (1983). DNA engineering: the use of enzymes, chemicals, and oligonucleotides to restructure DNA sequences in vitro. R. Williamson, ed. *Genetic engineering — 4.* New York: Academic Press.

Lear, J. (1978). *Recombinant DNA — the untold story.* New York: Crown Publishers.

Levine, J. (1986, November 3). The toughest virus of all. *Time,* 128 (18): 76-78.

Lemonick, M. D. (1987, November 9). The importance of being blue. *Time,* 130 (19): 82-83.

Lewin, R. (1983, December 23). The birth of recombinant DNA technology. *Science.* 222 (4630): 1313-15.

Newsweek, Inc. (1988, April 25). Small step for mice, large step for man. *Newsweek,* 111 (17): 58.

Ridenour, J. (1985, December 22). Ethics calls for wisdom more than knowledge. *The Grand Rapids Press,* p. D1-2.

Squires, S. (1985, December 23). Gene therapy: cure for nature's errors? *The Grand Rapids Press,* p. D1-2.

Thompson, D. (1987, April 20). The end of the beginning? *Time,*118 (16): 32-45.

Wade, N. (1977). *The ultimate experiment, man-made evolution.* New York: Walker.

Wallis, C. (1986, November 3). Viruses. *Time, 128 (18): 66-74.*

Watson, J. D. Tooze, J., and Kurtz, D. T. (1983). *Recombinant DNA — a short course.* New York: Freeman.

The Smith Family and Genetic Problems

The Smith family has a history of genetic problems. Mrs. Smith's mother has Alzheimer's disease, and her young child has Down's syndrome. Mrs. Smith wants to get pregnant and has been told by her physician that the possibility of having another child who is mentally deficient is quite high.

A pharmaceutical company investigating the relationship between Down's syndrome and Alzheimer's disease contacts the Smiths and asks if they are interested in participating in a controlled experiment involving gene splicing. The company representative tells Mr. and Mrs. Smith that with gene splicing steps can be taken to prevent Down's syndrome.

- How did the pharmaceutical company learn about the Smith family? Was there a breach of moral ethics? Is there an invasion of privacy?

- Do the parents have the right to submit the unborn child to experimentation?

- If the Smiths are paid money for participating in this experimental program, should they be required to put it in a trust fund for the unborn child?

- Could the gene splicing create other problems? If so, should the pharmaceutical company be held responsible?

- Should a legal document be executed to protect the unborn child from any unforeseen conditions that could result from gene splicing? If yes, what should be included?

- Should human beings be subjected to gene splicing? If so, who should be allowed to do it and under what conditions?

- If a couple is known to carry genetic traits that could be passed on to their children as inherited disorders, should they be required to submit to gene splicing when starting a family?

- If such a couple declines to have gene splicing performed, should they be allowed to have children? If not, how could such a rule be enforced?

- Would you suggest gene splicing to a member of your family if he or she was in a situation similar to that of Mr. and Mrs. Smith?

- Would you take advantage of the pharmaceutical company's offer if you were in the same circumstances as the Smith's?

3

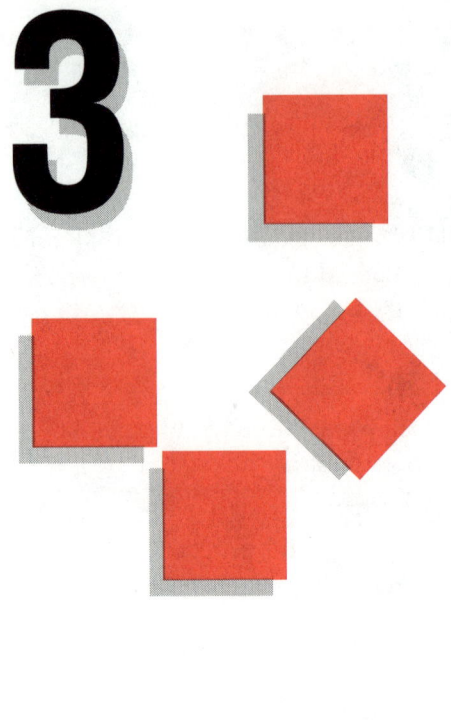

Patient Selection in Kidney Dialysis

Patricia Kearns Leitsch*

Objectives

After reading this chapter, you should be able to:

- Define the terms listed at the beginning of this chapter.
- Explain how the 100 percent Eligibility Rule affects patient selection.
- Explain two types of cost-containment procedures.
- Discuss how dialysis affects a patient's daily life.

Terms and Definitions

Artificial kidney dialyzer. The part of the hemodialysis machine that contains the membrane through which the blood passes during hemodialysis.

Chronic kidney failure/end-stage renal disease (ESRD). Destruction of normal kidney tissue that results in irreversible kidney damage.

Dialysis. Broadly defined as the movement of small molecules or particles from one side of a semipermeable membrane to the other side. Specific to ESRD, the medical treatment developed to remove the water, salt, and waste products from the patient's blood supply when their kidneys lose the ability to perform this function.

Hemodialysis. A form of dialysis that uses an artificial kidney machine to remove fluids and waste products from the bloodstream.

Kidneys. The pair of bean-shaped organs whose function is to remove waste products such as urea, phosphate, potassium, and uric acid.

Peritoneal dialysis. A form of dialysis that uses the patient's peritoneum to remove fluids and waste products from the bloodstream.

Peritoneum. The thin, smooth membrane that lines the cavity of the abdomen.
Renal. Pertaining to the kidneys.
Semipermeable membrane. A natural or artificial layer of material that contains small pores or openings.
Uremia. Accumulation of constituents in the blood that are normally eliminated in the urine; results in a severe toxic condition.

---

*Patricia Kearns Leitsch
Occupational Education Assistant Professor, School of Education, University of Louisville, Louisville, KY 40209.

Introduction

The three main bioethical issues involved in selecting patients for dialysis are: (1) government funds; (2) cost-containment measures; and (3) the patient's "quality of life" issues.

In 1972, the federal government guaranteed payment for dialysis, thus making treatment available to all patients suffering from end-stage renal disease. But over time, the numbers of such patients increased substantially more that was anticipated, and the federal government had to deal with another set of issues:

◆ What criteria should be used to contain costs?

◆ How should federal funds be distributed?

In addition, researchers had begun to explore the negative effects of dialysis treatment on the psychological well-being of the patient.

Renal Function, Failure, and the Rise of Dialysis

Before 1960, **end-stage renal failure** was the cause of death for more than 55,000 individuals suffering from **end-stage renal disease (ESRD),** a condition in which the kidneys are unable to perform their normal function of removing waste products such as urea, phosphate, potassium, and uric acid from the body. The primary causes of renal failure are various kidney diseases, hypertension, and diabetes.

By 1960, the outlook for such patients improved dramatically as the result of the development of the treatment known as artificial kidney dialysis. The treatment is based upon the principles of natural dialysis. The human body's blood supply contains toxins and waste products as a result of metabolism and exercise. As the blood supply flows to the kidneys, the potential harmful materials are exposed to the kidney's semipermeable membranes. When the kidneys are functioning normally, the toxins pass through the membranes, or dialyze from the blood to the other side of the membrane, and into the kidneys. The toxins are then eliminated from the body in the form of urine.

Two types of artificial dialysis were developed and named by the method of access to the body's toxins. The use of arterial and venal blood supply is termed hemodialysis and was the first type of dialysis developed. Initially, access to the vascular system was accomplished by direct needle insertion. The limited number of times a blood vessel could be entered in this manner prevented the development of continuous long-term dialysis. The development of tubes (cannulas) permanently placed in the artery and vein made possible long-term access to the blood supply. Surgically created passages from the artery to the vein (fistula) were an improvement over the cannulas.

The process of hemodialysis requires the surgical placement of some type of fistula to provide access to the patient's blood supply. The patient's blood is pumped into the kidney machine (artificial kidney). The kidney machine has two main parts: (1) a dialyzer which acts as the semipermeable membranes of the kidneys, and (2) the dialysate fluids inside the dialyzer that contain the body's normal balance of chemicals.

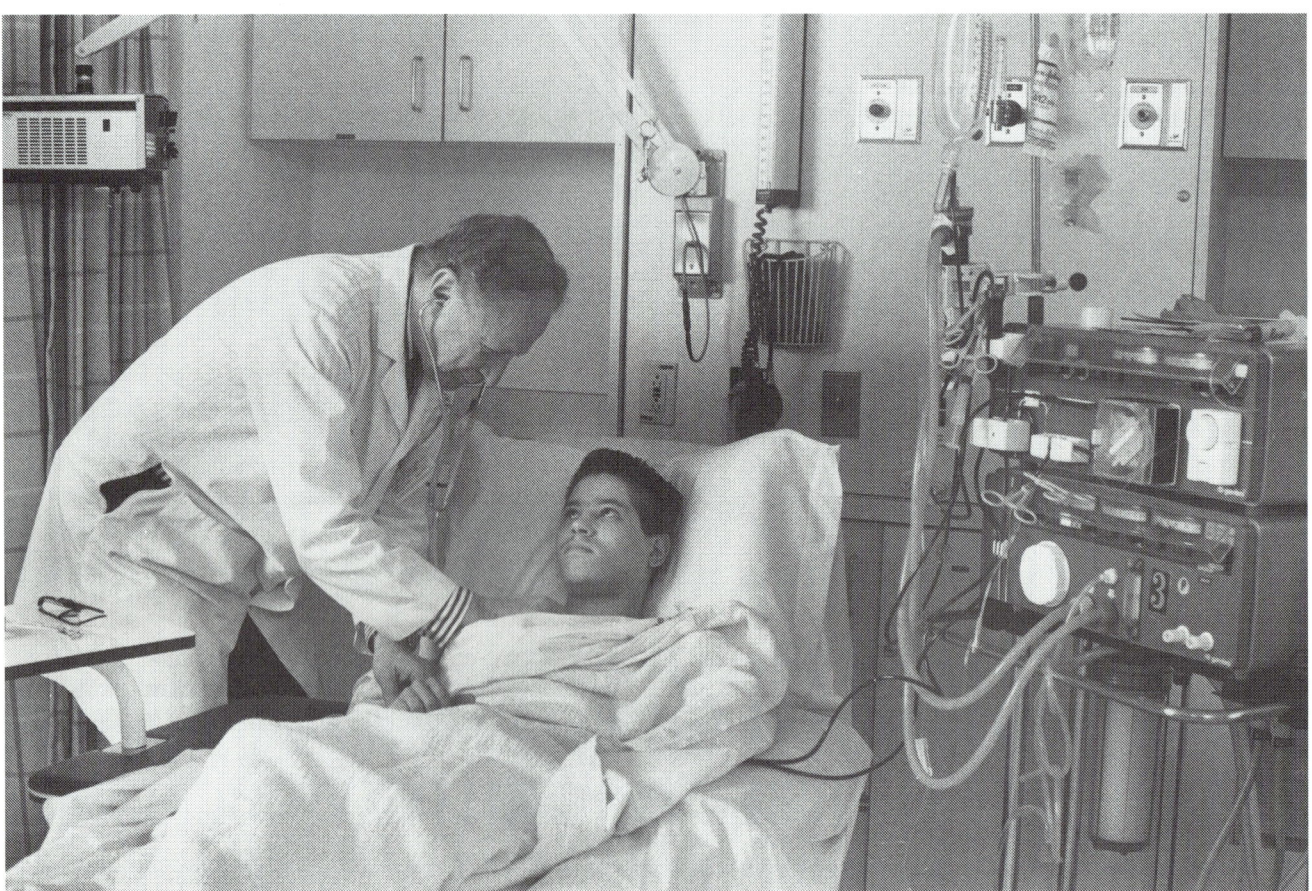

Patient receiving hemodialysis.

34

When the patient's blood supply, containing the toxins, comes in contact with the dialysate fluids, the toxins move from the blood into the dialyzer, thus cleansing the patient's blood supply. The cleaned blood is pumped back to the patient.

The second type of dialysis developed gains access to the body's waste products through a sac surrounding the intestines (the peritoneum) and is termed peritoneal dialysis. A permanent tube (a catheter) is surgically placed in the peritoneum. Dialysate fluid is injected into the peritoneum through the tube. The body's toxins pass through the semipermeable membranes of the peritoneal sac. After a half-hour, the fluids and toxins are drained from the abdomen through the tube, and the process is repeated for twelve to fourteen hours depending on the type of peritoneal dialysis chosen.

The annual cost per person on dialysis varies with the type of dialysis and with the location. Cost includes the insertion of access to the body's waste, dialysate fluids,

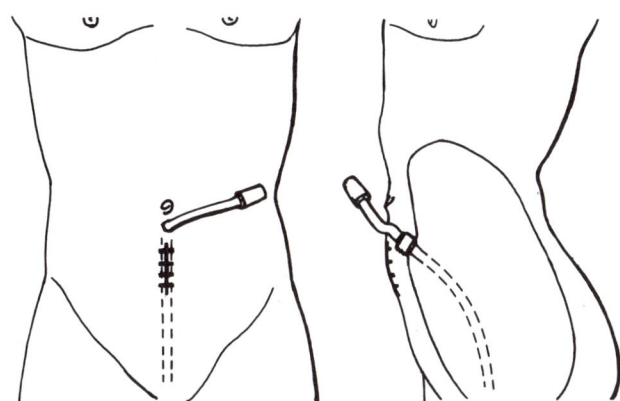

Placement of Tenchoff catheter in the abdomen; left 1/m frontal view showing site of insertion; and right 1/m placement into the peritoneum.

the dialyzer, and the personnel to provide treatment. Smith (1988) compared the cost of hemodialysis and peritoneal dialysis and estimated, based on 1983 dollars, annual costs of $23,344 and $21,429, respectively (excluding costs for additional medical problems). In 1989, Smith reported the costs per treatment for diabetic patients and nondiabetic patients on various forms of dialysis. One type of treatment included a combination of dialysis and the cost per diabetic was $40,779 versus $28,342 for the nondiabetic. Additional cost included the treatment of diabetes as well as the renal disease.

While both forms of artificial dialysis are effective in the removal of toxins, neither method is as efficient as the natural process. The human kidney is continuously removing the waste products as opposed to the scheduling required in artificial dialysis. For example, hemodialysis requires two to three treatments per week at an average length of three hours each. The patient experiences a sudden loss of toxins as opposed to a gradual loss and may experience fluctuations in blood pressure. In addition, dietary restrictions are imposed to avoid excess buildup of toxins between treatments.

Both forms of artificial dialysis present potential additional health risks. In hemodialysis, a small amount of the patient's blood remains in the dialyzer and can lead to anemia. Infections of the fistulae and peritoneal infections (peritonitis) are additional health problems.

Despite the inferiority of artificial dialysis, patients with ESRD must initiate and continue treatment in order to live.

As dialysis was developed, two major questions arose:

- How should patients be selected for dialysis?

- What type of dialysis treatment should they receive and where?

The answers were developed by the medical and political communities and are the source of the current ethical debate on dialysis.

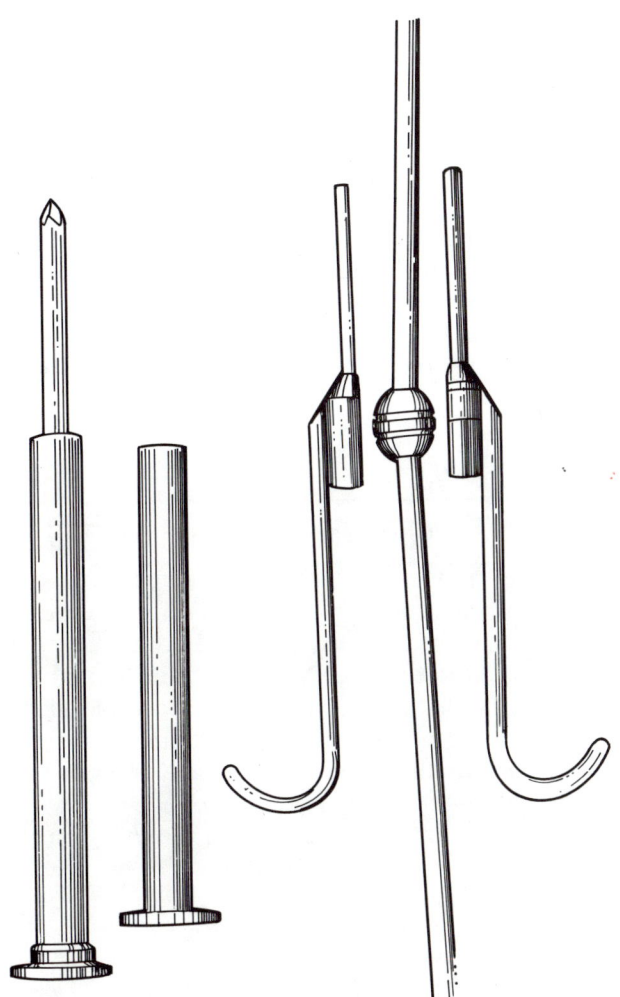

Example of a type of catheter used to access the peritoneum.

The United States ESRD patient selection process has changed as a result of various medical and political interventions. Initially, patient selection decisions were made by the medical researcher. During the developmental stages, the selection was based on the severity of renal failure and on whether dialysis was necessary for the improvement of the condition. By 1960 dialysis was available, but its use was limited because of the lack of sufficient facilities and finances. At that time, the average cost for dialysis was $40,000 a year. In an effort to use scarce resources efficiently, hospital personnel formed committees to develop and implement "nonmedical criteria to select which medically qualified candidates receive treatment" (Fox and Swazey, 1978). These medical committees became the gatekeepers of the scarce resources.

As the public became aware that the availability of dialysis was severely limited, pressure was placed on Congress to find a solution, based primarily upon humanitarian grounds. In 1972 Congress approved legislation that created the federally funded ESRD program.

Funding Issues

When Public law 92-603 became effective in 1972, the process of selecting dialysis patients and deciding on the modality of treatment was changed in fundamental ways. In essence the law said that virtually no one with end-stage renal disease would be denied treatment due to lack of facilities or funds. In order to accomplish this goal, Congress provided monies for dialysis through the Medicare system. With this broad definition of eligibility, 100 percent of the current population with renal failure was covered. The bill guaranteed 80 percent reimbursement to the center for dialysis treatment. In most cases, private insurance, state funds, or other agencies provided financial assistance for the remaining expenses. It is important to note that no other country has created this 100 percent rule. In most other countries, patient selection is still performed by committees and is based upon a public policy of treating only those patients that would benefit.

Public Law 92-603 encouraged and supported the proliferation of new centers. The hospital-based centers experienced the largest growth and number about 650. The for-profit, free-standing clinics were developed as a result of available funds and now total about 470.

As the number of centers grew, a change in attitude occurred in the medical community. Prior to the rapid expansion, dialysis centers were viewed as a scarce resource. Patient selection at that time was more deliberate, with emphasis placed on the good of the patient and society. As the number of centers increased, the resources were viewed as being in abundance. With this shift in attitude, patients previously not considered for dialysis were selected for treatment. Decisions to initiate treatment became less deliberate, and many more new patients were placed on dialysis.

The effects of change in the patient selection process were both immediate and long term. The elimination of the selection committees and removal of the nonmedical criteria were accomplished first. Prior to the law, treatment was viewed as a privilege, but as the ESRD program grew, treatment became a guaranteed right.

Cost-Containment Issues

Public Law 92-603 greatly influenced the dialysis treatment decisions. When regulations were developed to implement the new law, a dual rate of reimbursement was established. The hospital centers were paid more per treatment than the free-standing centers. This decision was based on the argument that the hospital would treat sicker patients who required more medical services. This dual rate indirectly influenced the growing preference for hospital centers. Therefore, from 1973 on treatment site decisions were influenced somewhat by the available funds.

When the ESRD program was approved, Congress was unaware of either the numbers of patients or the amount of funds required. In 1972 Congress believed it was funding the program for about 12,000 patients at an

---

Choice for Dialysis

Two patients come to the new dialysis center to be accepted into the dialysis program. One of the patients is twenty-five years old and has just survived a life-threatening bout with encephalitis. As a result, one kidney has been removed, and now the remaining, severely damaged kidney is in renal failure. The other patient is seventy-three years old, has been on dialysis for ten years, and otherwise is in excellent health. Because of center cutbacks, only one of these patients can be dialyzed on a long-term basis.

Which patient would you choose and why?

annual cost of $250 million (Greenberg, 1978). With these initial estimates, both the medical and political professionals were willing to place all renal failure patients on dialysis. But in 1981 there were approximately 68,000 Americans receiving treatment under the federally funded program at a cost of $1.2 billion (Greenspan, 1981). Social Security officials project that the program's budget will exceed $6 billion by 1990.

The dialysis population has continued to increase beyond the projections. Smith (1989) reported a cost of $2.5 billion per year spent on ESRD. Part of the increase is due to the number of diabetic patients placed on dialysis. Currently, one quarter of the total dialysis population is diabetic. Malangone (1989) reported similar data with 18.4% of the sample diabetic and 18.2% unknown onset of ESRD. In addition, Malangone reported an average age of 51.6 and one-quarter of the sample was 60 years or older. The older population tends to present additional medical problems and will increase the total cost to Medicare for dialysis.

The 1978 and 1982 amendments to Public Law 92-603 were introduced in an effort to contain the cost of the program. Cost-containment measures were directed toward sites of treatment rather than patient-selection decisions. The 1978 and 1982 changes were intended to encourage the use of the less expensive mode of treatment. At that time, home dialysis cost between $8,000 to $12,000 per year, as compared with $15,000 to $30,000 for center dialysis. Not only was the goal not achieved, but the percentage of home dialysis patients declined from 40 percent in 1972 to the current 16 percent. There are two reasons that the amendments were unable to curb the rising cost. First, no incentives or enforcement provisions were included to encourage the use of home dialysis. Second, the 100 percent eligibility rule was not addressed.

The increase in the dialysis population is the primary source of the large growth in the total program cost. Therefore, the most efficient cost-containment measure would be to limit the number of new patients placed on dialysis. To date, neither the medical nor the political communities have been willing to publicly support this decision. The "What is the price of life?" question raised by the media and supported by the public has limited the number of people who would support a change in eligibility.

In addition, the statement that "$15,000 per year is a small price to pay for life" is difficult to address. Politicians are afraid of being responsible for the loss of the "right" to treatment. Medical personnel are reluctant to support changing the 100 percent rule because of financial self-interests of the existing personnel and centers. As long as funds do exist, the current delivery systems will continue to survive and profit.

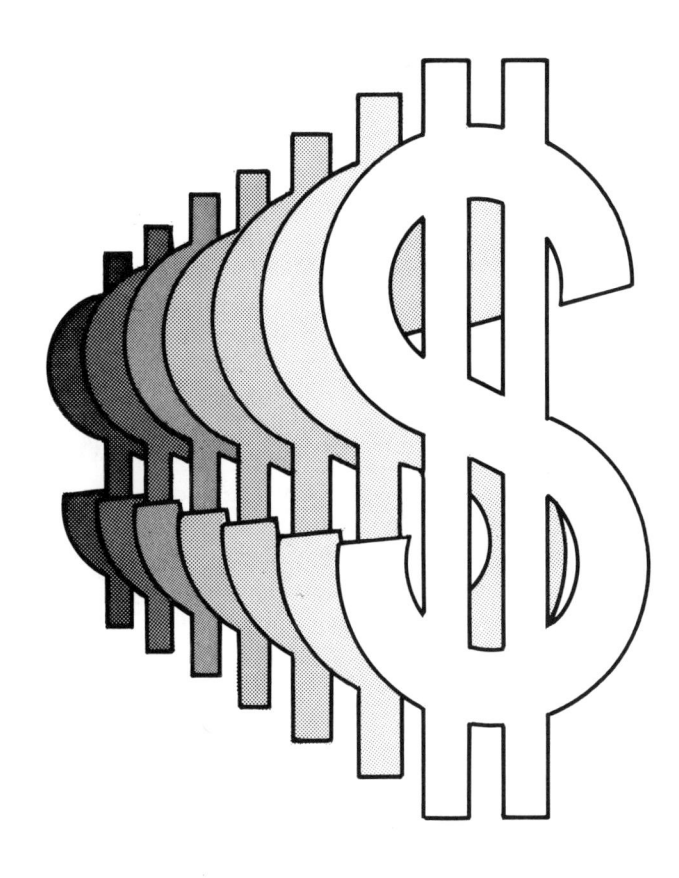

For these reasons, it is difficult to answer the question, "Can the 100 percent rule be changed?" If it could, the ethical considerations would include the need to develop criteria for patient selection. The return to the medical selection committees and criteria other than benefit to the patient should be considered in relation to the patient's quality of life.

A second, but less efficient, method of cost containment is the reduction of the daily operation expenses of the dialysis centers. To date, some cost-containment measures have been tried. The reuse of the dialyzers, reduction in trained personnel through the use of self-dialysis centers, and on-site mixing of dialysis fluid have been proven cost-efficient procedures. The effects these measures have on the quality of dialysis care and patient acceptance have not been studied. For example, formaldehyde is a chemical used in the dialysis process, but what do we know of the long-term effect of formaldehyde on the human system?

Containing the cost of the ESRD program is critical to the possible development of any other federally funded, disease-specific program. The rights of, and funds for, the ESRD patient are being weighed against those of patients with other life-threatening diseases. If costs are not contained, decisions may have to be made: what disease to fund, what kinds of treatments to fund.

Quality-of-Life Issues

Until the late 1970s no major research had been conducted to identify any psychological or sociological problems associated with dialysis. Since then, researchers have examined the problems of patients placed on continuous, long-term dialysis, using the broad topic of "quality-of-life" issues. Some of the identified psychological problems of dialysis patients are the same as anyone coping with any life-threatening disease, whereas others are unique to the dialysis patient. The dialysis patient's life depends on a machine that can be viewed as both threatening and necessary. Scheduling time for dialysis can be disruptive to family, work, and the social life of the dialysis patient. Side effects from dialysis and the development of additional medical conditions can damage the patient's sense of worth and self-esteem.

Each form of dialysis has a positive and negative effect on the physical and psychological well-being of the patient. The **hemodialysis** process has been studied for over 30 years and represents the better perfected treatment. The development of the fistulae has reduced the problems associated with maintenance of access to the vascular system. Improvements in the artificial kidney machine have increased safety for the patient. Years of data from monitoring patients on hemodialysis aid in the prevention of possible side effects of the treatment.

The major disadvantage of **hemodialysis** is the side effects created by the rapid loss of excess fluid and chemicals, such as headaches, cramps, fatigue, and hypertension. Since the patient generally receives treatment only two or three times per week, fluid and dietary restrictions are necessary. Hemodialysis involves some blood loss, and patients can develop anemia. Blood counts and transfusions are more common for hemodialysis patients.

Gertrude vs. High School Senior and Dialysis

Gertrude's life cannot be considered as a particularly easy one. She never knew her father.

She wore glasses and had a bad limp from a birth injury. She had few friends. The only friendly person in Gertrude's life was the next door neighbor who convinced Gertrude to consider a career in banking.

As a result of this person's urging, Gertrude got a job at the local bank and then went to college at night.

A year before she graduated from college, Gertrude's mother became ill with a heart condition and very dependent on Gertrude. The only good thing that seemed to be happening in Gertrude's life was that periodically she got a promotion. Her mother was getting progressively worse and no longer got out of bed. Her death and Gertrude's promotion to vice president of the bank came on the same day.

Six weeks after she buried her mother, Gertrude finds out that she has a kidney condition that requires dialysis. She checks into the local medical center for treatment.

At the same time, a senior in high school also requires dialysis. His name is Jack. He is an honor student and a hero to most of the students in school. He joined the football team when he was a junior and was immediately successful as a quarterback. In his senior year he was elected captain of the team and led the team to a successful season. At the last game he was injured and when examined by the team doctor was found to have a condition that requires kidney dialysis.

The hospital in this small community has the capability to take care of only one person requiring dialysis.

Which one should be selected and why?

Peritoneal dialysis is currently available in two forms: **ambulatory peritoneal dialysis (CAPD)** and **continuous cyclic peritoneal dialysis (CCPD).** CAPD and CCPD are both a home-based form of treatment and present the least amount of restrictions and burdens for the patient and family. Dialysis can be performed overnight, thus freeing the daytime hours. A patient can learn to operate the machine quite easily and may dialyze alone without fear of machine failure.

The major advantage of peritoneal dialysis is that it apparently reduces the side effects created by hemodialysis. This is due to the fact that with the former treatment the patient's chemical changes take place more slowly, and the body does not need to adjust to rapid change. Two major disadvantages of this mode of treatment are that the patient runs the risk of infection and that it is more time consuming. Depending upon the form of peritoneal dialysis chosen, the time for treatment ranges from four one-hour treatments for seven days a week to nightly dialysis of ten to twelve hours duration. As technology improves, the possibility of developing peritonitis is reduced. The problem of time will remain.

Dialysis treatment in the centers is given by trained personnel, and all equipment and supplies are provided. Patients are placed on a regular schedule that usually consists of two or three visits per week at an average length of three hours each. Center dialysis attracts patients for many reasons. The treatment is provided by trained personnel instead of family or friends. With treatment provided outside the home, some patients can lead a more normal life within the home. A major deterrent to accepting center treatment is the time spent away from home or work.

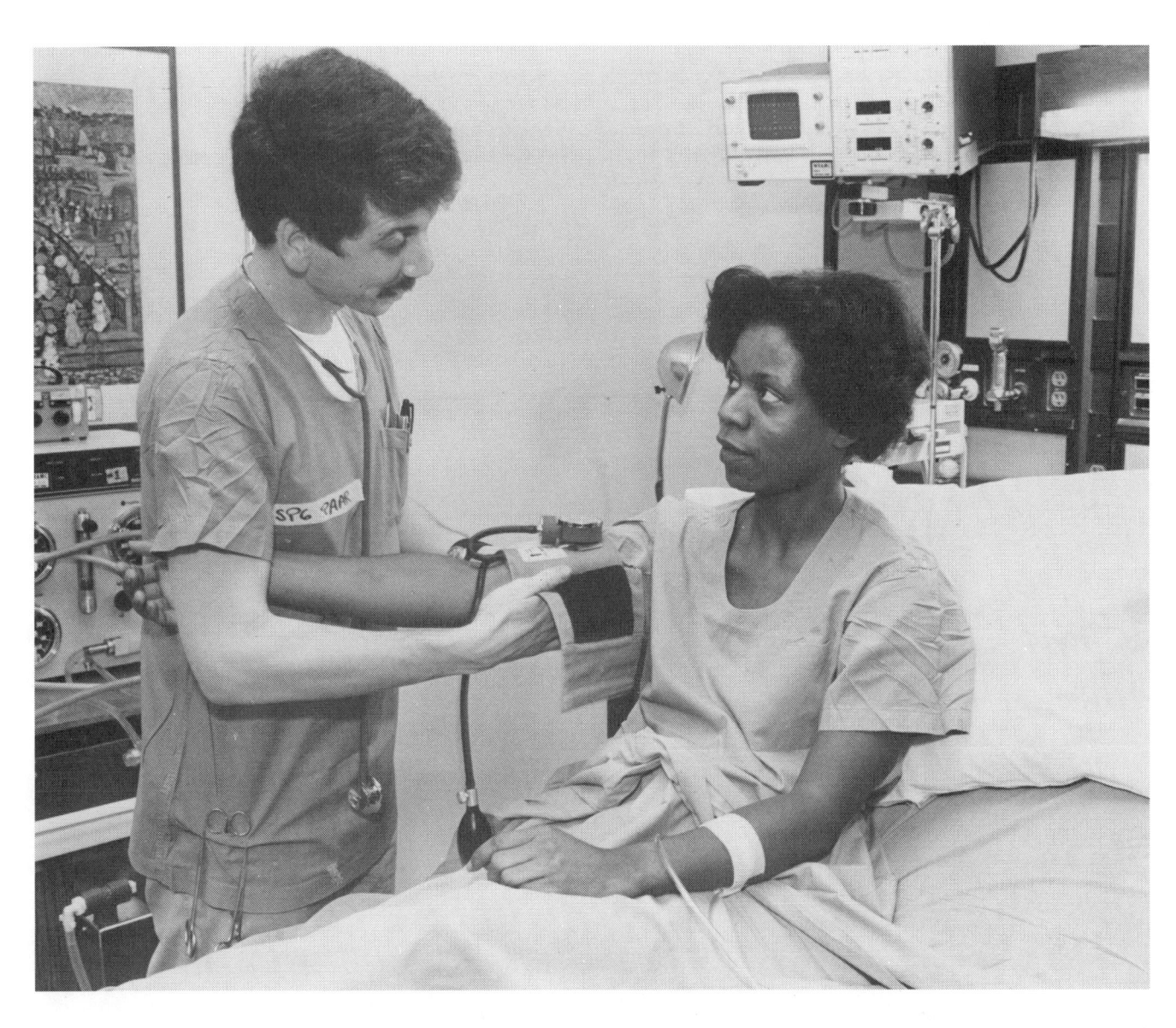

In contrast to center dialysis, **home hemodialysis** is provided by the patient's family and friends. The patient and responsible party must complete extensive training in the procedures of the treatment and equipment maintenance. Home dialysis patients must maintain and store all equipment and supplies needed for the treatment. This mode of treatment has one severe drawback: the responsibility placed on the family. The procedures and equipment require constant and intelligent attention. Breakdowns and problems will occur during treatment. Most lay people are not willing or able to assume this responsibility. In addition, they are often unable to provide "medical" treatment to their loved ones, preferring to defer to the trained professional.

At the present time, medical research has not proven that any one type of dialysis is superior or that a particular site is preferable. The decision about type and site of treatment should be based on the physician's experience and the patient's needs. The patient's physical condition and social and psychological needs should be matched with the side effects and constraints of each type of dialysis.

If the quality-of-life issues were to enter into the patient-selection decision, the appropriateness of the decision would improve. The staff must decide if the patient can tolerate the physical, psychological, and social adjustments required of someone on dialysis. The medical personnel must be willing to grant a negative evaluation and not recommend treatment. If the decision to begin dialysis is made, the constraints of type and site of treatment should be matched to the psychological needs of the patient and family.

The quality-of-life issue gained additional importance after a study by Neu and Kjellstrand (1986). They found that, in an 18-year period, 22 percent of all ESRD deaths were due to discontinuation of treatment. The decision to terminate treatment was made by the patient or the family and was made more often by older patients who had complicating degenerative diseases. The authors suggest that withdrawal from treatment will become more common in the future. These and other findings have generated ethical issues concerning the patient's right to terminate treatment and die. Additional research is needed to answer these new issues. Who should be involved in the decision-making process? Currently the decisions are being made by the patient or family in cases where the patient is incompetent. In addition, the decision to terminate treatment is being made on a case-by-case basis. Standards need to be established for deciding when to terminate dialysis.

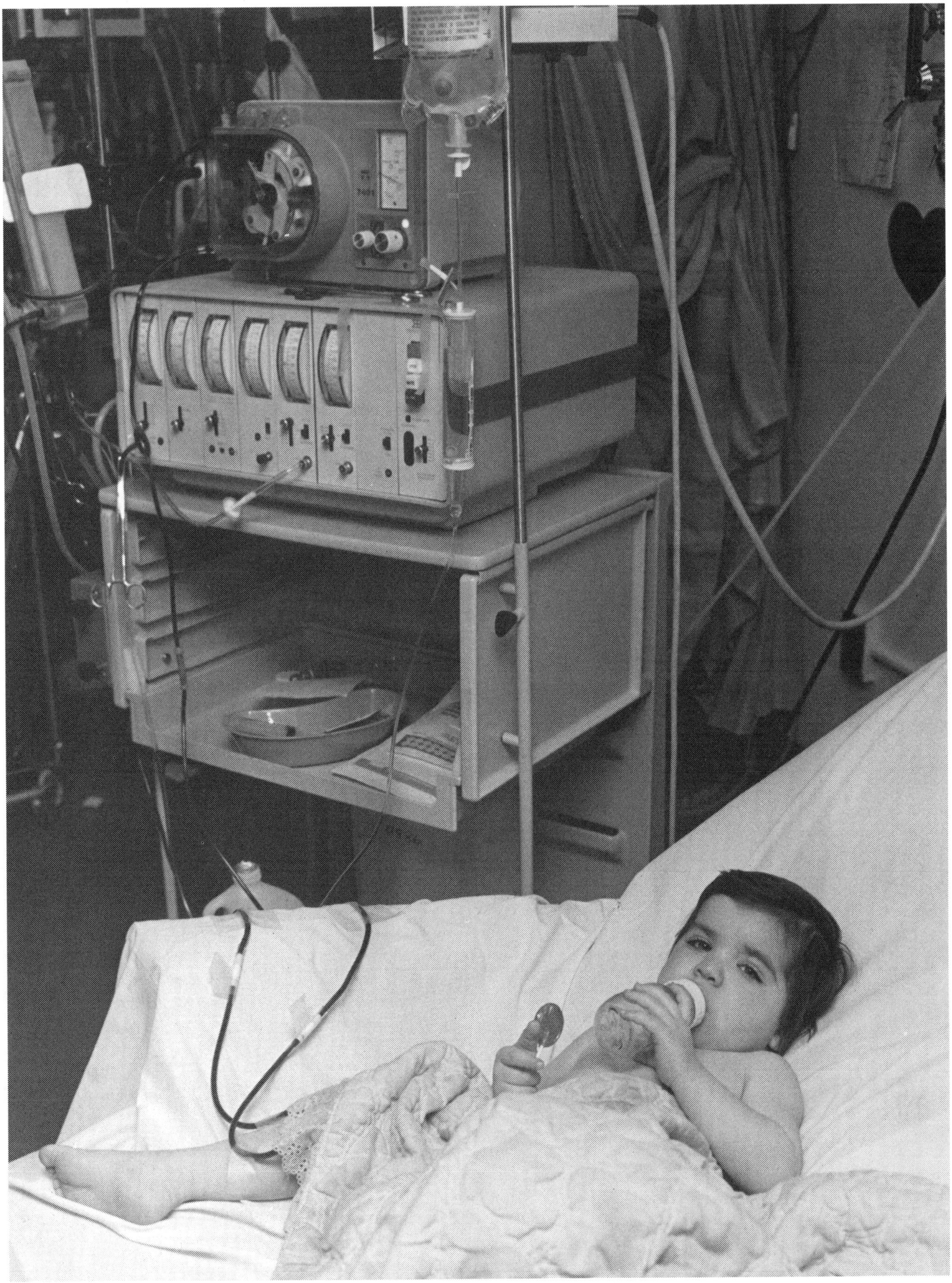

Summary

The ethical questions involved in selecting patients for dialysis are complex and interrelated.

Prior to the development of artificial dialysis, patients with renal failure or ESRD had no form of treatment available. With the development of the artificial kidney machine, the process of removing waste products from the blood supply could be accomplished. Currently, two forms of dialysis are available. Hemodialysis utilizes the vascular system to access the patient's waste products and peritoneal dialysis utilizes the peritoneum. In addition, both forms are available at centers staffed with trained medical personnel as well as for home use utilizing family and friends. To date, no form or site of dialysis has been proven superior.

Initially, patient selection was based upon medical criteria with the final decision made by committees composed of medical personnel. In 1972, Public Law 92-603 was passed and provided federal Medicare funds for all patients with ESRD. Eighty percent of the cost for dialysis was covered and the remaining 20% charged to private insurance. When Congress passed the 100% eligibility rule, the number of people and total cost were severely underestimated.

New dialysis centers were built to accommodate the increased number of patients who could afford treatment. As more centers were developed, more patients were placed on dialysis which increased the costs to Medicare. Congress made several attempts in the early 1980s to contain the cost of the ESRD program. The attempts were not successful due to the lack of incentives provided. Some centers are attempting to initiate cost-containment measures, but their long-term effects upon the patient's physical and psychological well-being have not been studied.

Representatives from medicine, government, and the general public need to address the 100% eligibility rule for patients with ESRD for two reasons. The current costs of ESRD stand at $2.5 billion annually and increase yearly. Secondly, other life-threatening diseases are competing for the dollars in the ESRD program.

Serious attention should be paid to the quality of life for patients with ESRD. The number of patients who voluntarily discontinue dialysis is increasing. In addition, the psychological problems facing the dialysis patients need to be addressed.

Cited References

Fox, R. C., and Swazey, J. P. (1978). *The courage to fail.* Chicago: University of Chicago Press, p. 208.

Greenberg, D. S. (1978). Legal politics. *The New England Journal of Medicine,* 298 (14): 1427-28.

Greenspan, R. E. (1981). The high price of federally regulated hemodialysis. *Journal of American Medical Association,* 246: 1901-11.

Malangone, J. M., Abuelo, J. G., Pezzullo, J. C., Lund, K., and McGloin, C.A. (1989). Clinical and laboratory features of people with chronic renal disease at the start of dialysis. *Clinical Nephrology,* 31 (2): 77-87.

Neu, S., and Kjellstrand, C. M. (1986). Stopping long-term dialysis: an empirical study of withdrawal of life-supporting treatment. *The New England Journal of Medicine,* 314 (1): 14:20.

Smith, D. G., and Wheeler, J. R. (1988). A comparison of charges for continuous ambulatory peritoneal dialysis and center hemodialysis. *Journal of Clinical Epidemiology.* 41 (9): 817-824.

Smith, D. G., Harlan, L. C., and Hawthorne, V. M. (1989). The charges for ESRD treatment of diabetics. *Journal of Clinical Epidemiology, 42 (2): 111-118.*

Additional Bibliography

Fox, R. C. (1981). Exclusion from dialysis: a sociological legal perspective. *Kidney International,* 19: 739-51.

Inglehart, J. K. (1982). Funding the end-stage renal-disease program. *The New England Journal of Medicine,* 306 (8): 492-96.

Lowrie, E. G., and Hampers, C. L. (1981). The success of Medicare's end-stage renal-disease program. *The New England Journal of Medicine,* 305 (8): 434-38.

Oberly, E. T., and Oberly, T. D. (1979). *Understanding your new life with dialysis: a patient guide for physical and psychological adjustment to maintenance dialysis.* Springfield: Charles C. Thomas.

O'Brien, M. R. (1983). *The courage to survive: the life career of the chronic dialysis patient.* New York: Grune and Stratton.

Robinson, D. (1982, October). Kidney dialysis: A taxpayer's nightmare. *Reader's Digest,* Oct. 149-52.

Smirnow, V. (1984). Patient selection: has Orwell's 1984 arrived? *Dialysis and Transplantation,* 21: 237-38.

Van Stone, J. C. (1983). *Dialysis and the treatment of renal insufficiency,* New York: Grune and Stratton.

Alex, Amanda, and Dialysis

Two people are admitted to the kidney dialysis section of a suburban hospital. The hospital has a major problem. It can provide service to only one patient, yet both need dialysis.

Alex is a thirty-year-old salesman who has lived in the community all his life. He attended the local schools and married his childhood sweetheart when she graduated from high school. They have been married about ten years and have three children. Alex has had poorly controlled diabetes since childhood. He now has moderately severe visual impairment, which has been made worse by his periodic drinking and continual smoking. Alex knows that he should watch his diet carefully and not smoke or drink, but he has found it impossible to stop either habit. When his boss found out that Alex had to be hospitalized, he told Alex not to worry about anything. He told Alex that he has full medical coverage and that all his bills would be taken care of by the insurance company.

The other person admitted is named Amanda. She is a twenty-two-year-old junkie who is six months pregnant. She takes a variety of drugs and has veins that are in poor condition. Her family does not know her whereabouts, and Amanda refuses to tell their names to anyone. She did disclose that she had dropped out of high school in her sophomore year because she didn't like the subjects or the teachers. Amanda was picked up by the police and taken to the hospital because of her poor physical condition. The clinic doctor discovers the pregnancy and also that Amanda has a condition that would require kidney dialysis.

Although both Alex and Amanda need dialysis, only one of them can receive it. You are the only person to make the decision because it is a holiday weekend and everyone is away.

- What factors should be considered when making the decision?
- If one of the patients were a member of your family, would that make a difference in your decision?
- If one of the people had political influence or were related to someone who did, would that make a difference in your decision?
- Should society have to pay for the treatment if people can't afford to pay for it?
- Should the fact that neither Alex or Amanda has taken care of themself be reason enough to prevent them from getting the treatment?
- Suppose Alex's physician is chief-of-staff at the hospital and a friend of the family, whereas Amanda has a new, young physician. Would this influence who gets dialysis?
- Should age or gender be a consideration in deciding which one should get the dialysis treatment?
- What influence should a person's obligations, such as the responsibility for children, have on the decision?
- Would it make any difference if Amanda were not pregnant?
- Would being chosen for dialysis create pressure on that person to change his/her lifestyle?
- Considering that suddenly there were two people who needed to have dialysis, might not a third party have need of the treatment? Should these two be refused in order to wait for a more suitable candidate?

4

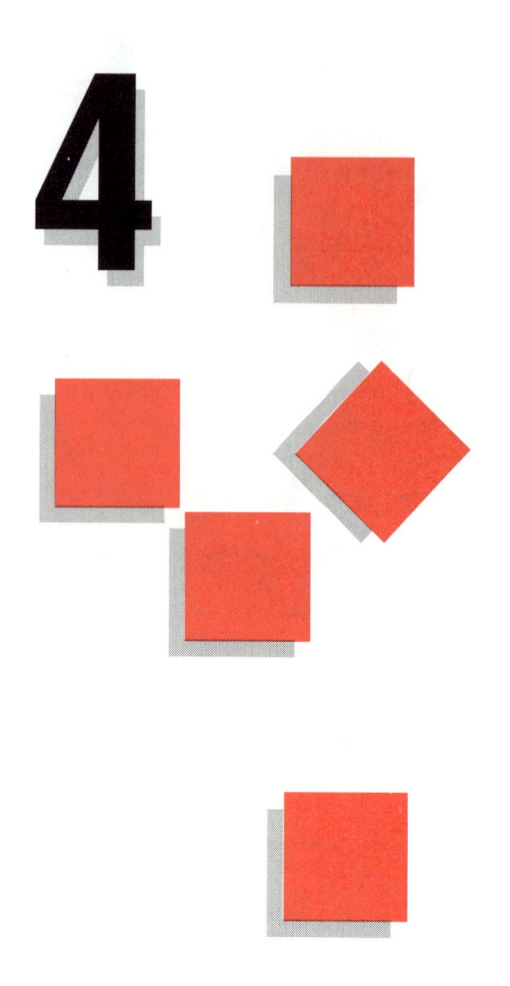

In-Vitro Fertilization, Embryo Transfer, and Surrogate Mothers

Mary Lou Park*

Objectives

After reading this chapter, you should be able to:

- Define the terms listed at the beginning of this chapter.
- Briefly outline the steps involved in in-vitro fertilization (IVF).
- Identify the costs of the IVF procedure, and reach a conclusion as to whether these costs are discriminatory against the poor.
- Give three ethical concerns about the surrogate-mothering process.
- Take a moral position on IVF and defend it.
- Detail the position of the Catholic Church on IVF and compare it with your family's and your own views.
- Describe three problems connected with using a surrogate mother to bear a child for another couple.
- Identify five options for having a child available to a couple who are childless for whatever reason.
- Describe the status of IVF and surrogate mothering as you foresee it to be in the year 2001.

Terms and Definitions

Artificial insemination. The introduction of semen into the genital tract of a female by other than natural means for purpose of impregnation.
Breach of contract. The breaking of a previously agreed upon course of action specified in a valid legal document.
Cloning. Asexual reproduction of cells, both plant and animal, by scientific means.
Cryopreservation. Controlled freezing of tissue such as sperm for usage at a later date.
Embryo transfer. Placement of the fertilized egg into the uterus for implantation after cell division has barely occurred.
Eugenics. The science that tries to improve the hereditary qualities of a race or breed.
Follicular recruitment. Stimulating the ovary with drug therapy, causing multiple follicles with ova to occur.
Gamete intrafallopian transfer (GIFT). Eggs are removed and mixed with sperm; the mixture is placed immediately in the woman's fallopian tube where fertilization by sperm occurs in the natural site.
Infertile. Unable to reproduce in a natural manner.

Informed consent. The act of agreeing to do something proposed or requested upon receiving information/education about the proposed act.

In-vitro fertilization. Fertilization of the mother's egg by the sperm outside the human body for purposes of transplantation into the uterus of the natural mother or surrogate mother.

Morals. Relating to principles of right and wrong in behavior. Considered a synonym of **ethics**.

Oocyte. An egg before maturation.

Oocyte recovery. "Harvesting," or gathering, the woman's eggs by passing an aspiration instrument through the abdominal wall to the ovary surface where mature eggs are collected from ovarian follicles.

Paternity. The state of being a father.

Reproductive capability. The ability to bear children or to reproduce.

Surrogate mother. One who bears a child for another usually for a fee in a prearranged agreement and who does not keep any rights to the child as the natural mother.

Sex-linked disease. An inherited condition that is sex linked, such as hemophilia, which occurs only in male children.

Theology. The study of religious faith, practice, and experience.

Tubal pregnancy. A situation where a fertilized egg remains to grow in the fallopian tube rather than passing to the uterine cavity for implantation and normal growth; the pregnancy is doomed to failure.

Wrongful life. A creation of life which is full of wrong, unjust, unfair, or injurious. A life which is without legal rights; unlawful.

---

*Mary Lou Park
Director of Health Services, Camden Central Schools, Camden, N.Y., and Adjunct Professor of Education, State University of New York, College at Oswego.

Introduction

The past twenty years have been a time of technological achievement and startling change which only the most imaginative science fiction writers hinted at half a century ago. Organ transplants, gene splicing, artificial hearts, prolonging life with high-tech equipment, and "pulling the plug" are all developments that threaten long-established beliefs and societal behavioral patterns. In-vitro fertilization is another example of the unprecedented capacity on the part of science to initiate, preserve, and destroy life.

In-vitro fertilization, or making "test-tube babies," and now the newer procedure, gamete intrafallopian transfer (GIFT), represent but two scientific triumphs that have raised profound moral, ethical, and legal questions. For the childless couples who have been able to achieve pregnancy via IVF, GIFT, or surrogate mothering, their babies are miraculous. To have a child of ones' own has created a booming billion dollar infertility business with an increasing number of daring new technologies and puzzling questions. This chapter explores the variety of questions raised and the processes involved in in-vitro fertilization, specific concerns, and pertinent legal materials.

Giant Strides over the Past Twenty Years

In-vitro fertilization (IVF), meaning "conception in a dish," refers to the fertilization of an egg **outside** the human body. Although we commonly say that this process creates **test tube babies,** that term is a misnomer, because the baby is not grown in a test tube! To be successful, the process must also include **embryo transfer (ET)** into the prospective mother's womb or uterus. IVF-ET is still thought to be experimental medicine. Physicians consider it a service of last resort for certain couples who wish to have a baby of their own because:

- it is very time-consuming
- it can be emotionally draining
- it can become very expensive

the success rate is low (While success rates are improving, the likelihood that any particular couple will end up with a baby is in the range of 9-12.5%.)

IVF-ET was first reported more than twenty years ago for not only human but ten different species of mammalian oocytes (eggs). The first living child born of this method was a girl baby Louise Brown, born in England in 1978. The doctors who performed the procedure, Stepcoe and Edwards of Cambridge University, immediately became world famous. The Brown family has since had another baby in this way.

By 1986, there were more than 150 clinics performing IVF around the world, with Scotland, India, and Australia considered pioneers. Totally, 3,700 IVF pregnancies had been reported at that time, and of that number about 2,000 births occurred. IVF had become increasingly common but was not necessarily accepted by all persons as a legitimate medical technique. In fact, IVF and other like procedures are still considered to be experimental medicine and not health insurance reimburseable.

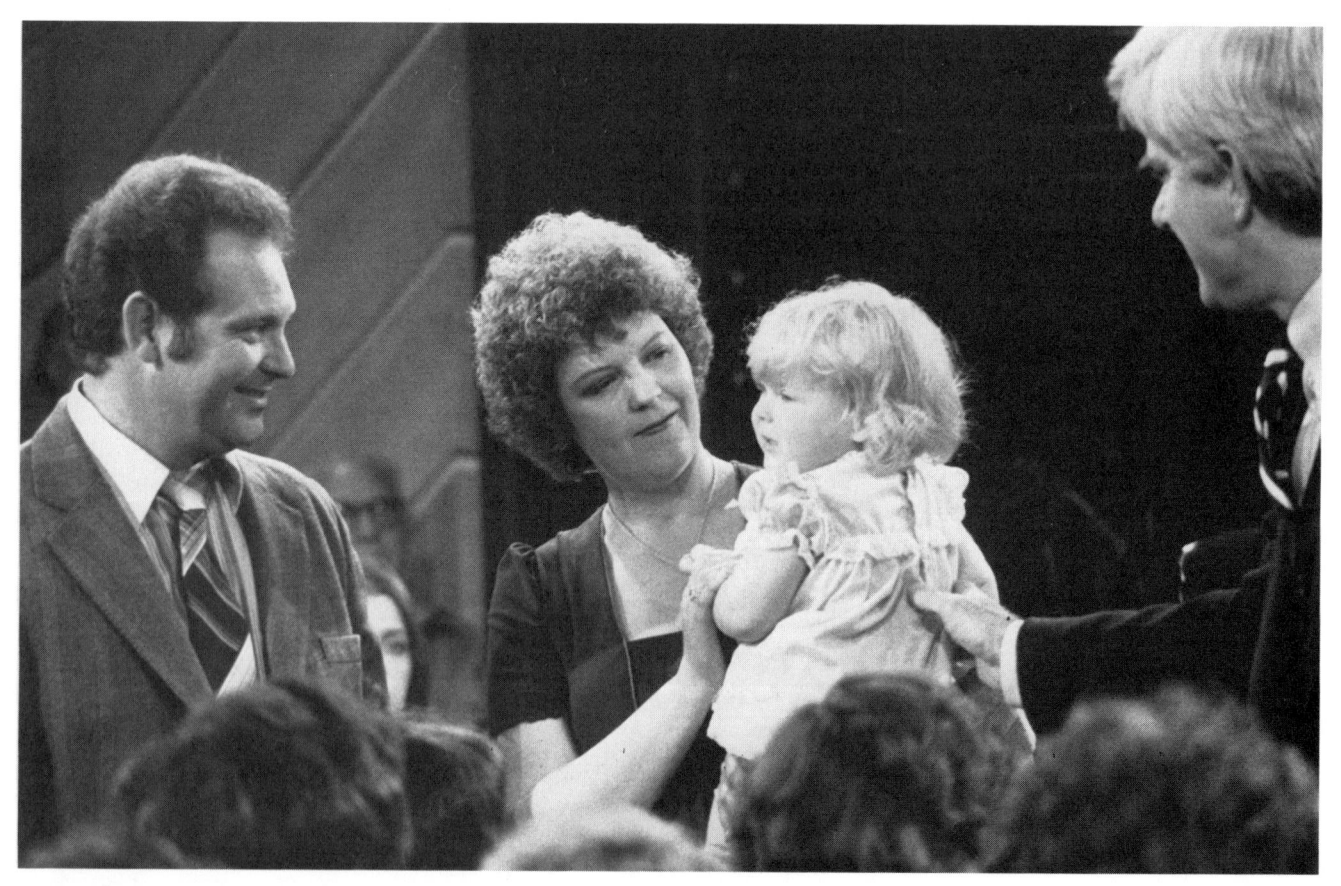

Louise Brown, the first IVF-ET baby.

In the United States, all clinics try to keep up with the Joneses, a medical couple who set up a clinic in 1978 at the Eastern Virginia Medical College in Norfolk upon their mandatory retirement from Johns Hopkins University. As a result of their work, the clinic had its first successful pregnancy/take in 1981 with the first live birth a few years later.

By 1989 in the United States, some 200 centers performed IVF, GIFT, or both along with other infertility solving procedures in a field still unregulated by federal or state governments. GIFT or gamete intrafallicular transfer is a fairly recent procedure developed in the United States. It is used for less serious infertility conditions such as endometriosis (an overgrowth of cells lining the inner uterine wall) or low sperm count. GIFT places treated sperm and retrieved eggs, which have been mixed together, in the fallopian tube by way of a catheter. Fertilization and pregnancy can then take place normally.

Success Rates of IVF and GIFT

Given the low percentage of births, one could ask, "Why bother to do this procedure?" The primary goal of IVF is to help couples to have children of their own, couples who have no other choice. It is indicative of the demand that one of six (approximately 2.4 million) American couples are infertile. The primary cause of the infertility is blocked fallopian tubes preventing eggs from reaching the uterus to be naturally fertilized and implanted. Secondary causes continue to be low sperm count and endometriosis. The advances in medical technology give these couples a chance to bear children (see accompanying box). In fact, IVF and GIFT have helped some 5000 U.S. couples to conceive and bear children. The only other real alternative is to adopt, but there are fewer babies to adopt owing to the increased use of contraception and abortion procedures. Although the in-vitro and intrafallopian processes are new and only have a 11-13% success rate, they offer hope where none had previously existed.

Success rates for IVF are increasing. Statistics for the Norfolk clinic show about 220 subjects by June 1986. These resulted in thirty-eight pregnancies, of which nine pregnancies resulted in babies born.

A federal report conducted by the Subcommittee on Regulation, Business Opportunities and Energy and Representative Ron Wyden (D-Oreg.), in cooperation with the American Fertility Society, obtained unbiased information about the performance of infertility clinics. In 1987, couples who tried a single IVF procedure have had an 11 percent chance of having a baby. Those who tried GIFT had a 13 percent chance. According to the report, success rates improved in 1988. The data for that year covered 1,661 pregnancies showed that IVF couples have a 12.5 percent chance of giving birth; the GIFT participants have odds of close to 20 percent. Success rates at infertility clinics vary widely from zero to 21% or higher.

Eight Ways to Have a Baby

1. Natural
2. AIH
3. AID
4. IVF — AIH — ET
5. IVF — AID — ET
6. SM — AIH or NIH
7. SM — AID
8. SM — Donor Egg — AIH

Key:
- AI = artificial insemination
- AID = artificial insemination by a donor
- AIH = artificial insemination by husband
- ET = embryo transfer
- IVF = in-vitro fertilization
- NIH = natural insemination by frozen sperm of husband

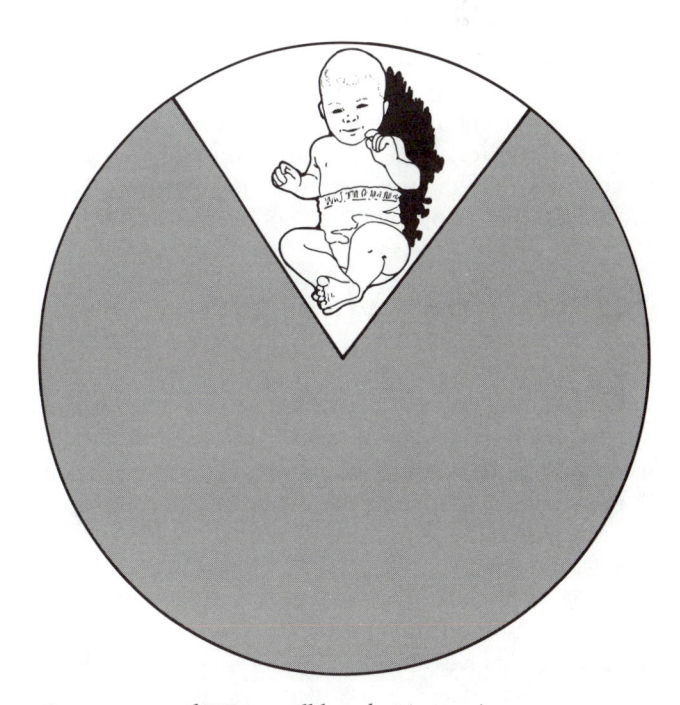

Success rates of IVF are still low, but improving.

The Process of IVF-ET

The process of in-vitro fertilization and embryo transfer involves six steps, which are presented in the accompanying chart.

The six steps are closely tied to the natural menstrual cycle. Great care is taken with each step, given that most women attempt the procedure just once owing to its high cost — in both financial and emotional terms.

An explanation of in-vitro fertilization steps (see accompanying box) is as follows. An injection of a gonadotropin drug is given to the woman which will stimulate many ovarian follicles to form (Step 1). Each will contain an ova or egg which will be harvested (Step 2) by laparoscopy under general anesthesia. The abdominal incision and instruments are the same as those utilized for "band-aid" or sterilization surgery. Each follicle is sucked out in order to obtain the egg which, after grading, is placed in a special laboratory medium or solution (Step 3).

Following incubation for 6 hours, a large number of sperm is added and left with the egg in the incubator for 18 hours. More than one egg or embryo may be incubated with sperm. After 22 hours, the eggs are examined for cell division (Step 4). At the point when there are two to four nuclei, the embryo is placed into the fundus or top of the uterus via catheter 2-3 days after recovery (Step 5). The recipient must keep her feet up for three hours and then stay in bed for 1-2 days. Pregnancy monitoring (Step 6) is done via a hormone blood level test (progesterone) and a blood test for pregnancy on days 24-26. On the 28th day either a pregnancy is diagnosed or menses begins.

About 15 to 20 percent of IVF births are twins and another 3 percent are triplets. Incidences of miscarriage are also higher, and tubal pregnancies are not uncommon. Given the experimental nature of the procedure, such happenings are not unexpected.

In-Vitro Fertilization

IVF-ET STEPS	CYCLE DAY
1. **Follicular recruitment.** from birth mother or surrogate. Woman is given gonadotropin drugs to stimulate multiple follicles.	3-10
Ultrasound is used to monitor follicle growth.	7-10
2. **Oocyte recovery (egg harvesting).** Laparoscopy is done under general anesthesia. Each follicle is aspirated to obtain a mature pre-ovulatory oocyte.	10-12
3. **Incubation.** After grading, an oocyte is put into insemination medium and incubated for 6 hours. 25,000 - 50,000 sperm (donor or husband) are added and left with egg for 18 hours.	10-12
4. **Embryo growth.** Embryo is observed for pronucleus formation. Fertilization is successful if polyspermia (2 pronuclei) has occurred. Eggs are left for 22 hours. Oocytes should have two to four cell embryonic development.	11-13
5. **Embryo transfer.** This step is done 48-72 hours after recovery. Deposited into fundus of uterus. Recipient keeps feet elevated for 3 hours and then bedrest for 24-48 hours.	12-14
6. **Pregnancy monitoring.** Progesterone blood level test.	19
Blood test for pregnancy.	24-26
Pregnancy or menses.	28

Surrogate Mothers

By definition, the act of serving as a surrogate mother involves bearing a child for another. While the word **surrogate** means a **substitute,** keep in mind that in most instances of surrogate mothering, the surrogate has provided the egg and is, indeed, the natural/biological mother.

Surrogate mothering requires a coordinated effort by medical personnel, mental health professionals, and legal representatives. If this is not done properly, there can be a prima facie malpractice case. Justification for surrogate mothering revolves around the fact there have been few, if any, laws that allow or disallow the practice. Furthermore, surrogate mothering is protected by the legal right to privacy and by the fact that there is a fundamental right to procreate — even if a couple has to go outside their marital union to do this.

Potential surrogates undergo a three- to six-hour consultation. It is essential that they are emotionally stable. Ninety percent of all potential surrogates are rejected. In screening, the reviewer looks for those who have had children and are mentally and emotionally sound. They must understand that the child will not be theirs. Candidates go through a medical exam, and some genetic matching is done. The cost for artificial insemination is $30,000; the cost for in-vitro fertilization is $40,000 to $100,000. The usual contract specifies that the surrogate receives $12,000 as well as medical expenses. Life insurance is provided, and every expense is covered: travel, maternity clothes, babysitting, and so forth.

Basically then, the process is this: a surrogate mother (SM) contracts for a fee to be artificially inseminated with the sperm of a man she often does not know or is implanted with the fertilized embryo. The SM carries the pregnancy to term and then gives the child to its natural father and/or mother. In so doing, she relinquishes all parental rights. The natural father's wife adopts the baby, and the birth mother's rights end.

Rachel

An example of surrogate mothering is found in the Bible: Rachel, wife of Jacob, used her slave Bilhah to bear Jacob's child when Rachel's own barrenness prevented her from doing so

Genesis 30.1-7:

When Rachel saw that she bore Jacob no children, she envied her sister; and she said to Jacob, "Give me children, or I shall die!" Jacob's anger was kindled against Rachel, and he said, "Am I in the place of God, who has withheld from you the fruit of the womb?" Then she said, "Here is my maid Bilhah; go in to her, that she may bear upon my knees, and even I may have children through her." So she gave him her maid Bilhah as a wife; and Jacob went in to her. And Bilhah conceived and bore Jacob a son. Then Rachel said, "God has judged me, and has also heard my voice and given me a son"; therefore she called his name Dan. Rachel's maid Bilhah conceived again and bore Jacob a second son.

Use of a Surrogate Mother

Sam and Sue have been married for five years and are trying to have a baby. Because Sue's fallopian tubes are blocked, she cannot become pregnant naturally. The couple has tried to have a test tube baby but have not been successful.

Now they are considering a surrogate mother. Sam is not interested in adoption. He wants his own child. It was his idea to use a surrogate mother, but Sue doesn't like it. She is concerned about the legal issues involved with such a relationship. She also fears that she will not feel the same about her child if it is born of a surrogate mother. She has shared her worries with her mother and finds that the rest of her family have similar concerns. When Sue gets up her courage and tells Sam how she feels, he laughs at her. He says that the only problem he can see is that the church will not christen the baby.

How can they work out a compromise?

Cryopreservation

Cryopreservation techniques of sperm and egg/embryos are a reality here and abroad, and have gained acceptance in recent years. Long a common practice in animals, it has several advantages over the usual IVF-ET technique. Many oocytes can be collected, or harvested, and then fertilized within a single menstrual cycle. Thus multiple oocyte recovery procedures are not needed. After embryo development occurs, the embryo is frozen. In subsequent menstrual cycles, embryo transfer is repeated until pregnancy occurs.

The first pregnancy resulting from a fertilized egg being frozen, thawed, and implanted in the natural mother's uterus took place in Canberra, Australia in 1983. This took seven years of research *and* a million dollars, but it did increase the odds of successful implantation. If use of this process becomes more widespread, it is not inconceivable that there will be egg banks in the future. Eggs may be donated and frozen for future use by individuals other than the donor.

Ethical Concerns Regarding IVF and SM

The public is interested in IVF and surrogate mothering, and the media coverage reflects this interest. In September, 1984, *Time* magazine ran an article, "A Legal, Moral, Social Nightmare," which caused quite a stir with its discussion of "huboons," baboons crossbred with humans. Books such as Gena Corea's *The Mother Machine* arouse concern for the surrogate mothers who are "being devalued for experimental purposes." The Phil Donahue Show of July 17, 1986, was devoted entirely to IVF, SM, and the effects of these new ways to have a baby. These and other media presentations are testimony to the American public's interest.

It is apparent that there is hardly any legal precedent for IVF and SM. No laws exist regulating these practices. Nevertheless, the medico-legal implications are great, especially in regard to surrogate motherhood, inheritance, and the case of frozen embryos. The number of court cases dealing with IVF and SM continues to rise, indicating that regulation may be needed. Court actions are not unique to any one country, but they do appear more often where these procedures are frequently performed. Any court findings are immediately published in law journals as well as reported in the press. The news is reviewed all over the world.

A basic issue is whether access to IVF should be legally limited, for example, to married couples only. The courts have previously ruled on the question of single mothers and AI fertilization as inappropriate, saying that a child needs two parents.

As more and more cases come before the courts, answers will need to be found for such questions as "Whose baby is it?" "What are the rights of the child?" "What are the rights of the surrogate mother?" Excerpts of recent legal findings can give some insight on what is being reviewed at present.

Rights of the Embryo

In common law, early Christian teaching (modified) said that "life was regarded as commencing at the unborn infant's first movement in the uterus or when it quickened and was thus infused with soul," according to Smith in *Family Law* (quotation modified). Theologians have voiced more than one interpretation of when life begins, however. Certain factions hold that it commences at the moment of conception. In the December 1979 issue of the *Futurist*, the comment is made that since many ova fertilized through IVF do not survive attempts at ET, those people who feel that life begins at the moment of conception insist that IVF is "morally unsupportable." Is this then a form of murder? If so, the embryo must be a person with rights at this stage.

What about the trauma or permanent damage that could occur to the egg during the IVF process. Paul Ramsey, a professor of religion, is also concerned for the health of the child, claiming that the process may do irreparable damage to the child-to-be. In addition, the rights of the child may be breached, for the unmade child has not "volunteered" to help the scientist or the mother.

Take, as an example, the infant born of the IVF process who has a genetic defect or abnormality. Technically speaking, the child could sue the experimenter/physician and hospital for negligence. Damages for pain and suffering could be awarded, perhaps as a case of **wrongful life**. The fetus/infant did not ask to be born; therefore, the infant's rights were violated.

R. Scott, in the *Australian Law Journal*, asks whether informed consent should be given by all participants involved in IVF. This requirement negates the process from taking place, for the embryo cannot give informed consent.

Theologians and philosophers alike probe the impersonal aspect of IVF, asking if this procedure can be considered human procreation. Is it only a means of simple manufacture accomplished by the laboratory? Some ask where is the concern for the personalization of the process and the sexual act as evidence of love? And how does this affect the integrity of the family unit when a SM, donor egg, or donor sperm is involved?

There was an additional concern in 1979 for possible abuse of human embryos: the danger of cloning and of creating human/animal hybrids. After girl baby Brown's birth, the U.S. Department of Health, Education, and Welfare's Ethics Advisory Board studied this aspect of IVF and ET. This board concluded that the embryo is entitled to profound respect, but that this does not necessarily encompass the full legal and moral rights attributed to persons. The law has to this day refused to recognize the moment of fertilization as the time when legal rights are conferred. This secular position contrasts strongly with that of the Catholic Church.

Position of the Catholic Church

In a statement by Pope Pius XII in 1956, he rejected IVF as absolutely immoral and later Pope Paul VI issued an encyclical entitled "Human Vitae" which banned all contraception. More recently, in March 1987, the Vatican released documents, approved by Pope John Paul II, that outlined the church's teachings on human reproduction.

Entitled "Instruction on Respect for Human Life in Its Origins and on the Dignity of Procreation," the documents condemned surrogate motherhood, test tube births, and experimentation on human embryos, including efforts to predetermine sex. A sterile couple's decision to have a child through in-vitro fertilization was deemed not an act of love but "an egoistic act." The forty-page statement rejected all modern technology that could either interfere with the process of conception or influence the development of the embryo.

Reaction to the documents around the world ranged from approval in Brazil, the world's largest Catholic country, to a vow of resistance in Ireland, which is predominantly Catholic. Heads of pioneer IVF programs in Kildare and Dublin said that the programs would continue and that the Vatican statement would not stop infertile couples from seeking medical help in order to have babies. In Lille, France, the faculty of that city's Catholic University said that they would seek "clarification" from the Vatican. The faculty was responsible for the first test tube birth in a Catholic hospital in September 1986. Only married couples had been used in their program, which took the wife's eggs and the husband's sperm.

The Vatican's reaction to medical innovations seeking to reverse sterility was considered to be tougher than expected. It clearly said that the church would not accept conception achieved without a sexual act between spouses. Time will tell the effect of the document upon individual behavior, whether it is that of Catholic scientists, medical personnel, church-run hospitals, and/or the individual.

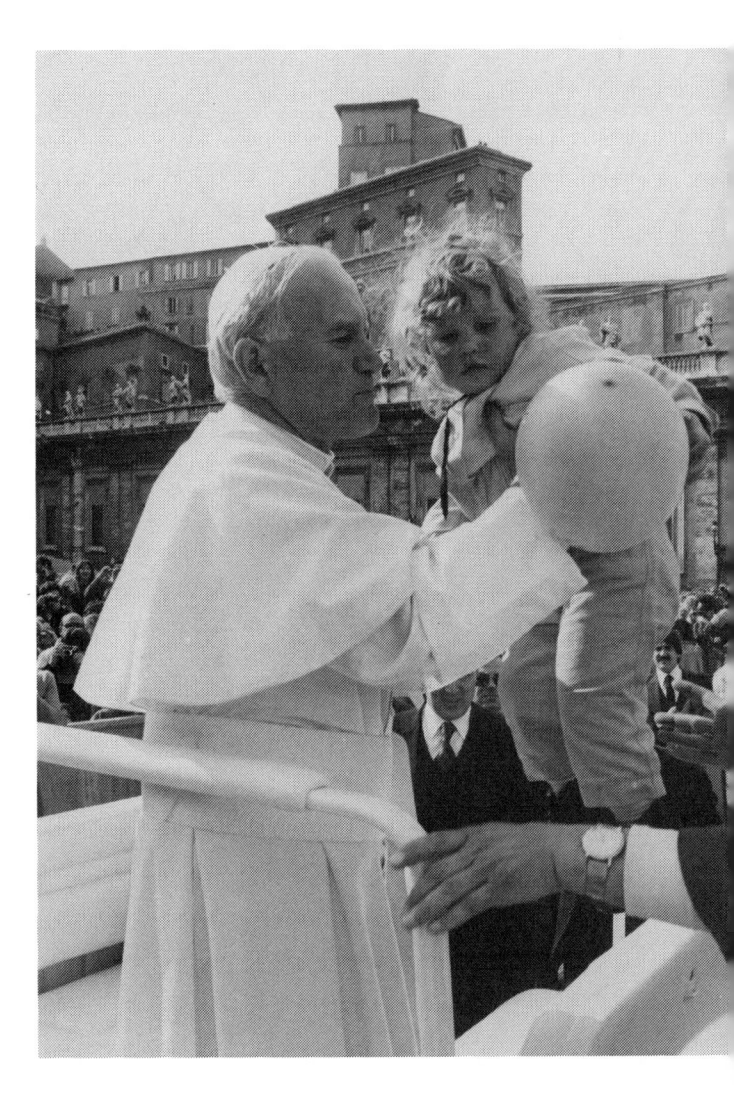

Eugenic Manipulation

H.D. Krause, writing in *Family Law*, worries about eugenic manipulation and the chance of scientists controlling human evolution. Suppose an abnormality is discerned during the embryo stage, and the embryo is destroyed. This is the first step toward deciding which fetuses are genetically worthy of life and which are not. Krause believes it is unethical to make such decisions.

In the *Saturday Review* of April 1972, Caryl Rivers writes of other concerns such as only having babies of one sex. On the plus side, one could in this way eliminate certain carriers of sex-linked diseases, but on the negative, boys would far outnumber girls as the more desired sex.

Frozen Embryos and Legal Rights

The case of the Australian frozen embryos generated more legal decisions about the rights of the embryo. Mrs. Rios was a thirty-seven-year-old who had had three eggs harvested and frozen. One egg had been implanted but had not resulted in pregnancy. Her husband was fifty years old, infertile, and had agreed to artificial insemination of these eggs. Both were killed in a plane crash, and although they left a large estate, they had written no will. The dilemma was what to do with the two remaining frozen embryos? If implanted in a surrogate mother, would they be the heirs to the fortune? The issues were if the two frozen embryos had a legal right to live via implantation in a SM and if they were born, could they claim inheritance rights to the Rios' estate?

One court ruled that the embryos had no legal rights or claims to inheritance because they were nonentities. As a result, the embryos were removed from storage and destroyed. Since they were not viable, no criminal liability was involved.

In another Australian court, it was decided that frozen embryos in situations like the Rios' *should* be implanted. The surrogate adoptive parents are the legal parents. This decision stated that one cannot legally stop the fertilization of human eggs, but neither can one demand that it be done.

As a result of this case, four legal theories concerning embryos and their possible rights were formulated.

1. In order for the embryos to be viewed as personal property, they must have economic value. This could not be accepted in the Rios' case.

2. The frozen embryos could be treated as children, and a guardian could be appointed.

3. The embryos could be regarded as nonentities and so would have no rights.

4. A repositor could be appointed, who as trustee for the deceased could decide the embryo's fate.

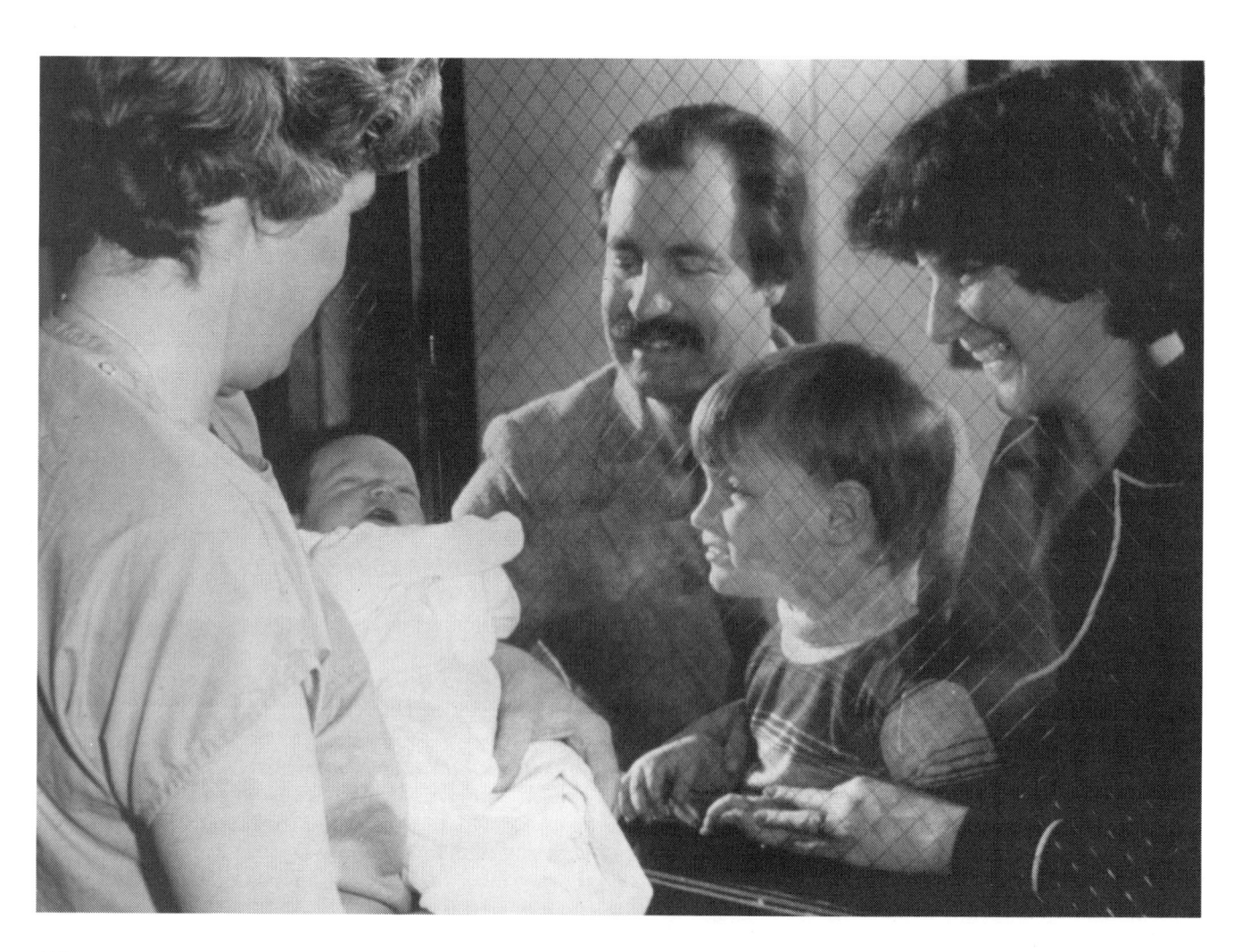

Financial/Commercial Aspects of IVF

The high cost of the IVF-ET procedure is a reality. It is experimental medicine, elective in nature, and insurance companies will not pay for it. Costs are paid by the client or with research monies at the clinic if they are available. In Australia, the expenses are about $5,700, which covers surgical retrieval of eggs. If a frozen embryo is used (cryopreservation is done in Australia) the cost drops to $2,800, for surgical retrieval has already been done. Costs at the Orlando Regional Medical Center in Florida were $4,100 in 1986, according to Dr. Gary DeVane of that clinic.

The Office of Technology Assessment recently released costs for the procedures as they exist in early 1989. They are as follows:

Diagnostic Workup	$3000 (up to)
Follow-up Treatment	8000
In-Vitro Fertilization	4000 to 6000
Gamete Intrafallopian Transfer	2500 to 6000
Freezing and Storage, Embryos	220 to 1800
Fertility Drug Treatment — 6-9 months	3668 average
Embryo Transfer	2500

Many people are concerned that IVF not only involves unjustified cost but will lead to unsavory commercialism. In response, medical practitioners have held that infertility is a serious problem that contributes to marital instability and may be a cause of mental health problems in many women; thus the treatment of infertility is of value. But what about the poor who are infertile and want children, yet cannot afford IVF?

Some people hold that the importance of biological parentage is overplayed and that the drive to have a child of one's own is given too much press; the limited funds available for health care in the United States would be better spent on the health of the poor or even on the prevention of venereal disease – a major cause of infertility. There may be an element of racism in IVF: if the infertile couple really want a baby so much, why do they refuse to take hard-to-place children of another ethnic or racial background?

Those wishing a "natural" child are willing to pay a lot in order to have one. The desire can become a consuming need. This could lead to a black market for donor eggs, as it has for babies to adopt. If there is a double embryo (as there often is), it could be cut in two for the value of the extra egg. It is not inconceivable that a donor could be recruited as a nonspousal source of sperm or eggs.

In *The Mother Machine* Corea speaks of the recruiting of women from Third World countries, such as in Africa, to serve as hosts for implanted fertilized eggs. Simple payment of room and board during the pregnancy would be a welcome bonus to one so poor. Any poor woman in the world could be exploited in this way.

Whose Baby Is It? The Dilemma of Surrogate Mothering

Surrogate mothering has generated many legal, moral, and ethical dilemmas. The practice has been challenged by those who consider it to be selling a child and hence illegal. Contracts involving the sale of children are contrary to public policy, in that the act may lead to a black market and charges of buying a baby illegally. The question revolves around the issue of whether the surrogate mother (SM) is providing a *service* or a *product*.

A variety of contract disputes have occurred. One instance is when the SM does not wish to surrender the child after giving birth and is accused of fraud or breach of contract. She may be threatened and give up the child out of fear. This may be coercion and not breach of contract. On the other hand, if the couple breaches the contract, the court awards damages. The natural mother can put the child up for adoption.

In another example: if the state has an artificial insemination law, the law can be a barrier for the natural father in establishing paternity. By law, the artificial insemination donor has no rights to the child and cannot claim to be the natural father; instead, the surrogate mother's husband (if there is one) is considered the child's natural father or the "legitimate issue" of that "father."

In California, the risk of losing money invested in the SM is real. The adopting father usually pays for maternity and living expenses of the SM. By law, any payment cannot be contingent upon adoption placement, whether a regular adoption or SM adoption. Once they have paid, parents cannot get any money back, since the funds are considered charity.

On occasion, the natural mother changes her mind because of an emotional attachment to the newborn. Under usual circumstance, the courts hold that the rights of the natural birth mother are paramount, and that the integrity of the family should be preserved. The family may be the only institution where one is loved, not for what one does, but for what one is. But to which family does the baby belong? To the natural birth mother or to the couple who made the arrangements? (See accompanying box on the "Baby M" Case.) And where will the baby be happier?

We have already touched on the possible danger of exploiting poor women who would serve as hosts for implanted fertilized eggs. By the same token, surrogate mothers by artificial insemination might choose this course of action because of their poverty. Surrogate mothers might be used for the convenience of the genetic father and mother, as when the latter doesn't want to deal with the discomforts of a pregnancy that might disrupt her career. There is much debate about these exploitive aspects of the SM process, as well as the legality of the contracts themselves.

The states must still struggle with the legality of surrogate parent issues and whether or not the contracts should be outlawed as a matter of public policy. E. R. Shipp writing for the *New York Time* news service (April 2, 1987) stated that "judges in New York, New Jersey, Kentucky, and elsewhere have continued to deliberate in a legal limbo, faced with biomedical advances and trying to make them fit into the moldy framework of laws on adoption, custody, and the granting of parental rights." At the same time, third-party parenting advocates hailed the original New Jersey court decision, saying that surrogacy is now here to stay. The appeals process muddied the issue however.

The Child of Artificial Insemination: Whose Baby Is It?

- The child's relationship to a married female artificially inseminated from donated sperm: The one who bears the child is considered the legal mother.
- The child's relationship to the donor of the semen when the ovum is fertilized by sperm given by donor or husband: The father is the legal parent if he consented to the insemination by his own or donor's sperm; by law, the donor must remain unknown.
- The child's relationship to an infertile female who receives the donation of an ovum. The ovum donor is out of the picture; the one who bears the child is the legal mother.
- The child's relationship to an infertile wife and husband who receive donations of both egg and sperm: They are the legal parents; donors are not. If a surrogate mother is used, she must turn over the child, according to English law.

The "Baby M" Case

No court action involving a surrogate mother has received as much attention as the "Baby M" case in Hackensack, New Jersey, in 1986-87. The dispute was centered on a woman who agreed to bear a child as a surrogate mother but refused to give up the baby after it was born. The key figures and scenario in the "Baby M" case are as follows:

- **Mary Beth Whitehead**, twenty-nine-year-old housewife who gave birth to a girl, on March 27, 1986, after signing a $10,000 contract to be impregnated with William Stern's sperm and be a surrogate mother. She refused to hand over the child, fled to Florida, and subsequently threatened to kill herself and the child via a telephone call to the child's father.

- **Richard Whitehead**, husband of Mary Beth, who supported his wife's decision and quit his job as a sanitation worker to flee to Florida with his wife and the baby.

- **William Stern**, forty-year-old biochemist who contracted with Mrs. Whitehead to bear a child for him using his artificially inseminated sperm. He and his wife had temporary custody of the child pending the outcome of the trial.

- **Elizabeth Stern**, forty-one-year-old pediatrician who planned to adopt the child when the surrogate mother gave up her parental rights. The Sterns undertook surrogacy because of their ages and because of Mrs. Stern's mild case of multiple sclerosis, claiming these were deterrents to natural birthing.

- **Baby M**, called Melissa by her father and Sara by her mother, who appeared unaffected by the situation according to evaluations by mental health specialists.

- **Harvey R. Sorkow**, the family court judge who was the first in the United States to decide on the validity of a surrogate contract.

- **Gary N. Skoloff**, attorney for William and Elizabeth Stern who argued that his clients were the more fit parents and that Whitehead had breached the contract. Skoloff is the author of a definitive three-volume textbook on the subject which is used in law schools and law libraries.

- **Harold J. Cassidy**, chief counsel for the Whiteheads, and **Randolf Wolf**, co-counsel. Neither were family law specialists. Wolf was adamant that this was a case of exploiting the poor for personal benefit.

Following a widely publicized court case, Judge Sorkow ruled that the father would be the better parent. Excepting the contract between the parties, he stated that this was a classic custody dispute where the judge was to determine what would be in the best interests of the child. The judge declared that the "right to enter into surrogate parenting contracts was protected by the 14th Amendment of the Constitution, which guarantees privacy and equal protection under the law (Syracuse Herald-Journal, 4-1-89)." The decisions in the Baby M case are pertinent only in New Jersey and were appealed.

"Baby M" turned three in March of 1989 and by that time sixty bills had been introduced in state legislatures and three in Congress to ban, regulate, or study surrogacy. The New Jersey Supreme Court in 1988 outlawed surrogacy for pay in the state and State Senator Catherine Costa had introduced a bill to regulate arrangements for surrogacy contracts. States that have declared surrogacy contracts void and unenforceable are Louisiana, Nebraska, and Kentucky. Surrogacy for hire is illegal in Florida but a woman can volunteer to bear a child for someone else and be paid for expenses. The American Bar Association has issued a blueprint for legalizing surrogacy which details approval by a judge of the pact before conception and that the egg or sperm would come from a married couple. Additionally, the surrogate mother would have up to 180 days to change her mind *after* conception. The ABA does not endorse surrogacy, however.

Baby M or Melissa lives with William and Elizabeth Stern in Tenafly, N.J. with one six-hour visit a week from her biological mother. Mary Beth Whitehead-Gould calls her Sara, the name on the child's birth certificate. Mrs. Whitehead-Gould divorced Whitehead and is now married to Dean Gould, father of her fourth and fifth children. Mrs. Whitehead-Gould did return the surrogacy payment of $10,000 to Stern. She has written with Loretta Schwartz-Nobel a book entitled "A Mother's Story" (published by St. Martin's Press) which begins with the birth and ends at Baby M's second birthday.

Gary N. Skoloff who was a lawyer for William Stern is among those who are supporters of surrogacy, saying that it should be legalized but should be well regulated. It is his belief that, once all the debates are finished, surrogacy will be legalized in a few states where all couples will go. It is his view that this will protect the children by statute and give them legal protection.

Summary

The joy of infertile couples who successfully gain a child through IVF and/or surrogate mothering cannot be denied. Medical technology is to be congratulated in making the couple's dreams come true. The difficulties appear to lie in the areas of theology, morality, and ethical behaviors and in the fears of some that misapplications can cause challenges to the accepted or traditional way of doing things.

Such new developments as genetic engineering, cloning, and manipulation of embryos have led to a fear of chimeras (monsters). Should IVF be stopped for fear of what the scientists may do next?

The question of the rights of the child and of the natural mother serving as surrogate must be resolved. The commercial aspect of the issue is not to be ignored, even though some deny that their motives are economic. Motherhood — traditionally as American as apple pie and hitherto unassailable — has now become a controversy in church, courts, clinics, and cottages.

The issues and problems will not go away and will multiply in the future. There is a great need for guidelines acceptable to all and for sound and objective counsel.

Cited References

Books, 60 bills spring from Baby M case. (March 12, 1989). *Syracuse Herald American* newspaper.

Krause, H. D. (1985, Fall). Artificial conception: legislative approaches. *Family Law Quarterly,* 19: 185-206.

Smith, II, G. P. (1985-86). Australia's frozen "orphan" embryos: a medical, legal, and ethical dilemma. *Journal of Family Law,* 24: 24-41.

Additional Bibliography

Cohen, B. (1984, Fall). Surrogate mothers: whose baby is it? *American Law Journal and Medicine,* 10: 243-85.

Dickens, B. M. (1985, Summer). Reproduction law and medical consent. *University of Toronto Law Journal,* 35: 255-86.

Discussion on bioethics (1984, July). *New Zealand Law Journal,* 237-44.

France, J. (1984, July). In vitro fertilization: a brave new world? *New Zealand Law Journal,* 234-36.

Frozen embryos: the constitution on ice. (1985, November). *Loyola/Los Angeles Law Review,* 19: 267-83.

Genesis retold: legal issues raised by the cryo-preservation of preimplantation human embryos. (1985). *Syracuse Law Review,* 36: 1021-53.

Hollinger, J. H. (1985, Summer). From coitus to commerce: legal and social consequences of non-coital reproduction. *University Journal of Law,* 18: 856-932.

In vitro fertilization: third party motherhood and the changing definition of legal parent. (1985, October). *Pacific Law Journal,* 17: 231-59.

Kennan, J. (1985, August). Science and the law — lessons from the experience of legislating for the new reproductive technology. *Australian Law Journal,* 59: 488-93.

Sloman, S. (1985, October). Surrogacy Arrangements Act, 1985. *New Law Journal,* 135: 978-80.

Surrogate parenthood — an analysis of the problems and a solution: representation for the child. (1986). *William Mitchell Law Review,* 12: 143-82.

The high cost of fighting infertility. (March 1989). *Changing Times* magazine.

What do infertility clinics really deliver? (April 3, 1989). *U.S. News and World Report* magazine.

A large number of medical and legal journals were consulted when researching this topic. Those printed materials of the most value are listed here. Valuable information was obtained from Dr. Gary DeVane of Orlando, Florida, and his inservice presentation sponsored by the Orlando Regional Medical Center's Staff Development Department in May 1986.

The Industrialist's Wife and Pregnancy

A *South American industrialist, father of six females, wants a son to carry on the family's name and to inherit the family business. He and his wife come to the United States, where his wife is scheduled for cosmetic surgery. It is a two-part procedure: the first operation will be the internal reconstruction of the vaginal vault and the second will be the removal of excess stomach adipose tissue (tummy tuck).*

The industrialist wants eggs to be removed during the first operation and then fertilized in the laboratory. The woman will be impregnated as a result of the fertilized test tube ovum being inserted during the second operation.

His wife has refused to have any additional children. The industrialist feels that once she learns she is pregnant she will carry the child to term. He has learned that a particular doctor has a very high success rate and wants him to arrange for the procedure. He offers the surgeon a very substantial sum of money for this service. He also stipulates that the wife not be told.

- Does a woman have the right to say whether she will be pregnant?

- Why does the industrialist feel his daughters cannot carry on the business, or if not the daughters, their husbands?

- Is the husband violating the marriage contract and his wife's trust by having this procedure performed without her knowledge?

- What will his relationship be with his wife should she discover his intrigue?

- If his wife dies as a result of this pregnancy, will he be guilty of manslaughter?

- What kind of legal recourse can or should the wife be able to take as a result of her husband's action?

- Suppose the fertilized egg is implanted in another person's body (surrogate relationship), should he tell his wife what has occurred, and if so, when?

- If a surrogate mother is used, what attitude might the wife and the six children have toward the baby?

- What are some of the relationships that might exist between the surrogate parent, the baby, and the industrialist and his family?

- What are some of the demands the surrogate mother could make on the industrialist and his family?

- What are some of the demands the surrogate mother could make on the industrialist, his family, and/or the physician in the future?

- If a male child is born to the surrogate mother and the industrialist dies, what legal problems could arise?

- Should the physician receive money for the covert aspects of this situation; if yes, when should the money be paid?

- How can the physician guarantee that all persons involved in this procedure, such as the lab technicians and nursing staff, will keep it confidential?

- Should physicians be allowed to perform an elective procedure that may cause physical and/or emotional harm to their patients?

5

Human Behavior Control: Realities and Possibilities

Ruth M. Patterson*

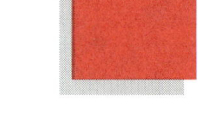

Objectives

After reading this chapter, you should be able to:

- Define the terms listed at the beginning of this chapter.
- Discuss various types of behavior control.
- State several important codes of ethics in the medical fields.
- List several examples of methods used to manipulate our physical and mental state.
- State the three R's needed today in relation to the study of bioethics.
- List several modern novels that describe unethical practices of behavior control.

Terms and Definitions

Behavior research. Research that deals with human actions.
Biomedical. Branch of medicine concerned with human beings.
Consent. Voluntary authorization.
Informed Consent. The right to know all about a procedure before agreeing to the procedure. Permission is given voluntarily after the person understands what will be done.
Manipulation. To control by unfair or insidious means, especially to one's own advantage.
Psychosurgery. Brain surgery employed in treating symptoms of the mind or mental processes.
Roulette. A gambling game in which players bet on the compartment in which a small ball will come to rest.
Subliminal. Existing or functioning below the threshold of conscious awareness.

Introduction

Has your behavior been controlled or altered today? Did you take prescription drugs or over-the-counter medications? Did you consume coffee, soft drinks, or chocolate for the caffeine lift? Did you purchase products that magazine or television advertisements manipulated you into purchasing? Do you ever wonder why your parent in the nursing home is so lethargic when you visit? Do you use a cocktail or sleeping pill to "unwind" after work? Newspaper articles describe suits filed against the CIA and the Armed Forces describing supersecret programs using people as living test tubes or chemical mixing bowls. Some of these "subjects" have committed suicide, but terrifying nightmares continue for many who still live. Look at the popular medical novels *Coma, Brain, Mindbend,* and *Outbreak* which describe behavior control for personal gain.

Great potential for harm exists in behavior control as well as ethical, social, and legal issues. With a central nervous system so complex that it exceeds the most sophisticated computer known to humans, the human animal is continually altering moods, thoughts, feelings, and behaviors. The President's Commission for the Study of Ethical Problems in Medicine and Biomedical and Behavioral Research reminded us that we are creating the kind of world we want to live in by the choices we make on these issues. Are we making odd choices when given the opportunity?

A powerful intermingling of medical science and the humanities is producing a crisis in health care today. Physicians and health care workers are moving into brave new worlds. Medical science is exploding with new ideas and ingenious new mechanical body parts, making the Bionic man or woman a real possibility. Technological advances, however, have outstripped our understanding of the ethical implications of these new discoveries. We can no longer hide from these issues but must confront them and make some choices. Dialogue between members of the health professions and moral philosophers must be ongoing. Drifting with the tide, or just allowing things to happen, is unthinkable, and we cannot afford to do this.

Altering the behavior, and thus lives of human beings, could be seen as a form of Russian roulette. Webster (1984) defines **roulette** as a gambling game in which players bet on the compartments in a wheel into which a small ball could fall when the wheel is turned. Webster, likewise, defines **Russian roulette** as an act of bravado consisting of spinning the cylinder of a revolver loaded with one cartridge, pointing the muzzle at one's own head, and pulling the trigger. Why are we so concerned with the bioethics of behavior control today? Is it because some types of behavior control may be compared with the idea of Russian roulette? When a human being is aware that ingesting alcohol, prescription or illegal drugs, or submitting to psychosurgery will alter the neurochemical balances of the body but does not know the extent or outcome of the altered state, the person can certainly be considered to be playing a form of Russian roulette.

---

*Ruth M. Patterson
Assistant Professor, Health Occupations Teacher Education Program, North Carolina State University, Raleigh, North Carolina 27695.

Physical and Mental Manipulation

Do we understand that magazines and television advertisers have been manipulating us to purchase items we do not desire, but items that our brains received messages to purchase? Do we understand that overmedication and the resulting lethargy facilitates management of large numbers of patients in nursing homes? Is it possible that the "nocturnal agitation" charted may be caused by patients desiring to use the bathroom and lack of staff to answer the call lights? Are we aware that we are putting a drug into our body when we need another cup of coffee or another Coca Cola to help us get through the day? How about the sleeping pill when we have insomnia and the cocktail after a stressful day? Do we take a mood elevator when we are depressed, and a Valium when we need to calm down?

Subliminal Messages

Key (1973) discussed subliminal messages, including actual magazine advertisements which had appeared in national magazines with hidden messages directed to an unsuspecting public. Dillingham (1987) wrote:

> "Subliminal programming has come a long way in the years since 1956, when a New Jersey movie theater, hoping to boost sales at the concession stand, flashed 'Drink Coca-Cola' and 'Eat popcorn' between frames of Kim Novak's image in the movie, 'Picnic.' Presumably, the theatergoers were not consciously aware of the messages, which appeared on the screen for just a fraction of a second at a time, but legend has it that soft drink and popcorn sales went up dramatically. The ruse was quickly denounced as unduly manipulative and Big Brotherly, and use of subliminals was banned in advertising."

Audiocassettes with self-help messages in subliminal form are a booming business today. While the public hears only relaxing music or simulated ocean waves, hundreds or thousands of tiny messages are encoded that help us lose weight, stop smoking, stop drinking, improve our self-esteem, relieve pain, succeed financially and much more.

Subliminal Advertising in Mexico

Garcia (1988) interviewed a Mexican father, Mario Tinoco, who was driving to work in Mexico City with his 11-year-old daughter when she said, "I saw the devil in that billboard." Tinoco pulled off the busy roadway to see for himself the horned head with satanic grin in the billboard advertisement. This instance of a subliminal message to an unsuspecting public sparked a nine-year passion for Tinoco, ferreting out and studying subliminal ads on Mexican television.

"It has been almost a full-time job because the airwaves are saturated with them," Tinoco says, surrounded by sophisticated video equipment, editing machines, and computers.

Tinoco explained that hidden messages evolved from symbols used by prehistoric man before languages. Since symbols are universal, manipulation can occur regardless of what language the viewer might be speaking. According to Garcia,

Mastery of hidden messages 'came into its own in World War II Germany under Goebbels, who was a master manipulator.' Moviemaker Alfred Hitchcock was a pioneer in applying hidden symbols with the new technology of television and films.

"'Hitchcock understood fear and tension. His trick was to insert a single skull image into a film sequence and heighten audience expectations and fear. He was a master at that,'" he says.

"Subliminal advertising in the United States has been prohibited by law for years. Not so in Mexico."

"With the aid of computers and an electronic editing machine, Tinoco and his staff can slow down and dissect ads frame by frame. What they have found hidden in some ads 'have been hairraising, incredibly sensual or simply outrageous.'"

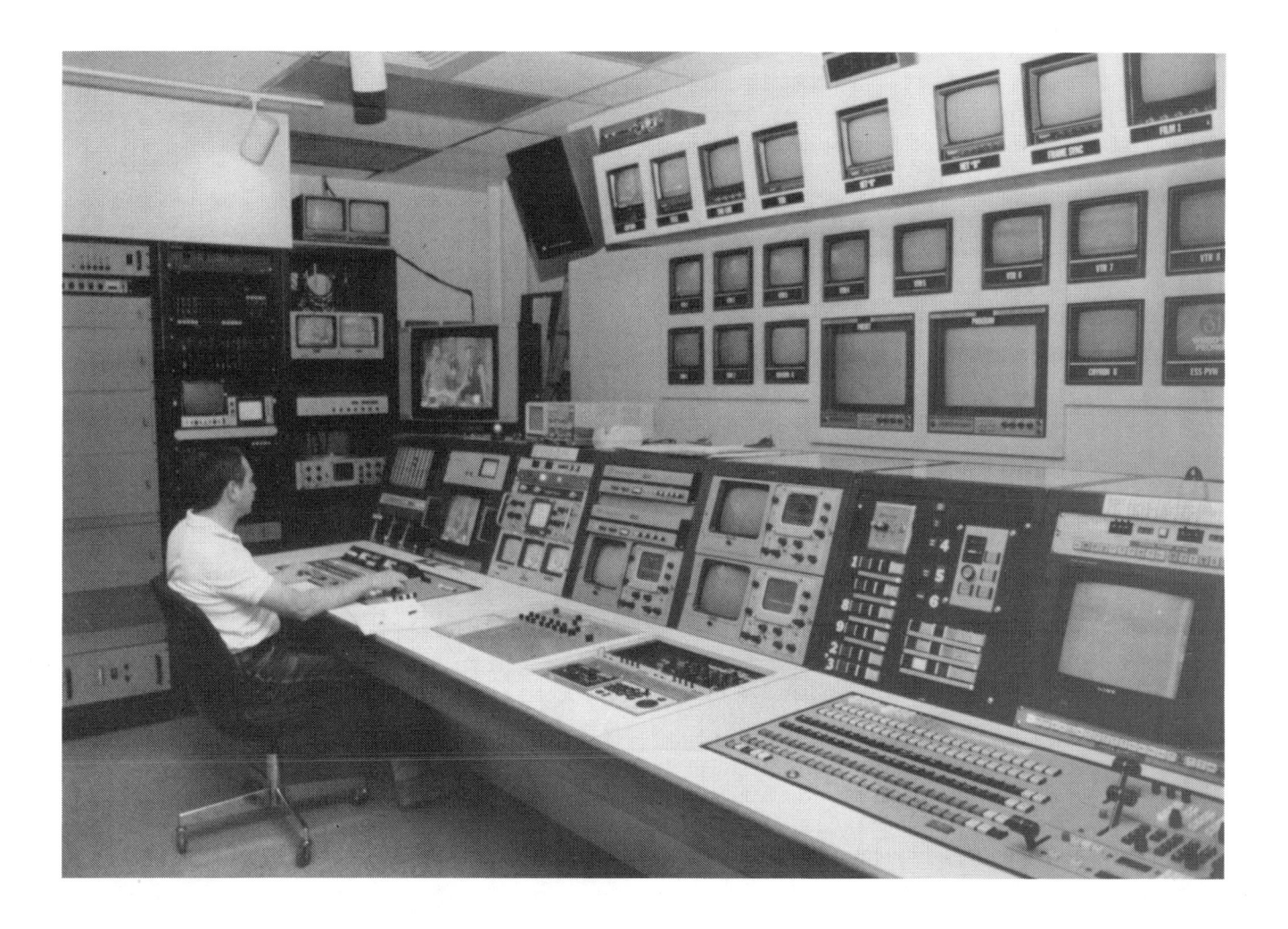

While the U.S. Federal Communications Code has banned subliminal advertising, there are no regulations governing subliminal communication. Subliminals are being played over public address systems to increase employee productivity, relieve anxiety at the dentist, and deter shoplifting in department stores. Some states are considering bills prohibiting the use of audio or visual subliminals in the workplace after growing public concern about unconscious manipulation is surfacing.

Grumman (1987) says that it is impossible to verify the contentions since subliminal messages are literally playing with the person's mind and that is not ethical unless the public asks for or consents to this behavior control.

Allman (1989), in a study on television and advertising, has concluded that normal advertising – typically $150,000 for production and more millions to air – is not actually paying off at the cash register. Emotions and cultural values sway the public more than rationale and statistics, according to his conclusions. Psychological research on the brain's reflex actions suggested loud noises and sudden movements of light would cause the eyes and ears to focus in the direction of the stimulus. (Note that commercials are always louder than programming.) Since subliminal symbols have been outlawed in U.S. advertising, knowing how or why the U.S. public makes a choice of items means greater profits to the advertiser.

A Dallas, Texas radio station ("Radio Station Runs," 1987) broadcast subliminal messages simultaneously with regular music at four pre-announced times in 1987 as part of the American Cancer Society's Great American Smokeout. The station's attorneys said the messages would not violate the FCC law because listeners were told in advance of the subliminal messages.

Psychosurgery

With all these frightening possibilities, however, one of the most serious methods of behavior control seems to be psychosurgery. With human brains more sophisticated than any computer, how can we dare tinker with mind-altering drugs or brain surgery with the idea of controlling the behavior of a human being? Providing relief from unrelenting pain or destroying a brain tumor might be reason to open the skull and destroy a tiny segment of the brain, but with only a slip of the scalpel or cautery, a valuable part of the patient's personality could disappear.

At any moment, 25% of hospital beds in the U.S. are filled by mental patients, more than the total for cancer, heart disease, and respiratory illness patients combined. (Goode, 1989, p. 60)

Dorothea Dix, the crusading schoolteacher who took up the cause of the mentally ill in the mid-1800s, would not believe the changes that have occurred with the advent of psychotropic drugs such as *Haldol, Mellaril, Stelazine,* and lithium.

Exposés of inhumane treatment and lobotomies which were performed on over 50,000 patients in the 1930s and 1940s were described by Andrews (1977). Stating psychosurgery's potentially dangerous outcomes, Andrews uncovered this surgery being performed for everything from hyperactivity in children to alcoholics and drug addicts. Foes of this procedure likened it to "doing surgery with your eyes closed" because of the possibility of loss of a valuable part of the patient's personality during the destruction of brain tissue.

The President's Commission (1983) reported deep concern for the implications of informed consent when patients are participating in research, quasi-experimental procedures, or medical treatments. "A California court has ruled that psychosurgery is so harmful and intrusive that it is not to be performed on mental patients until a hearing is held to determine the voluntariness and competency of the consent" (Andrews, 1977, p. 43).

- Who will determine the "potentially violent" mental patient who is sent for psychosurgery?
- Who will decide that psychosurgery is a "cost-effective" method of managing large numbers of mental patients?
- Who will make certain that the patient has freely consented to the procedure and understands the possible consequences?

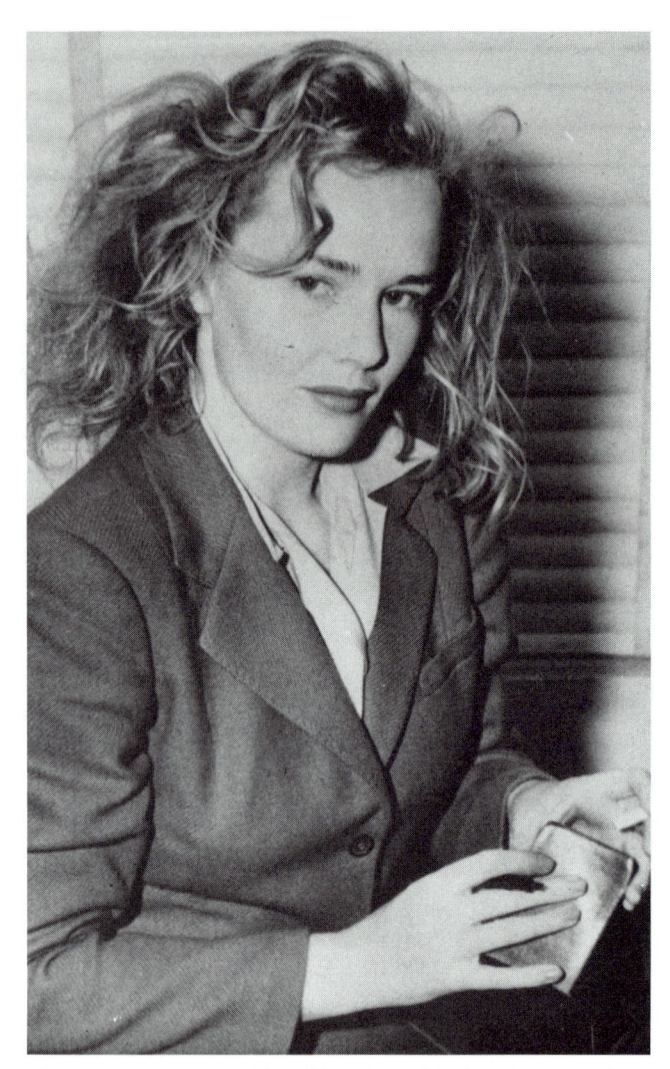

Frances Farmer, a victim of inappropriate psychosurgery?

- Could this procedure ever become a scandalous method of controlling society?

Only a dozen states grant mental patients the right to refuse psychosurgery at this time (Andrews, 1977).

Psychotherapeutic Centers

Psychotherapeutic Centers advertise in our daily newspapers that they will help persons cope with the stresses of living. They offer phobia programs for compulsive eaters, programs aimed at the compulsive-obsessive personality, or programs to help you stop smoking. They no longer require a medical referral to accept patients for behavior modification.

Drug Use

Allegations of inappropriate use of *Ritalin,* a drug given to hyperactive children, have led to numerous lawsuits nationwide. This drug, which acts on nerves in the frontal lobe of the brain, can alter attention span, excitability, and impulsiveness of children and must be prescribed with caution.

More than a decade after a federal study found serious abuse of drugs in nursing homes, many patients still are being drugged just to make them easier to care for. The study ("Many patients") showed that more than forty percent of nursing home patients are given drugs just so nursing home staff can control them more easily, especially on weekends when the homes are apt to be short-staffed. Often the drugs were given without the consent of the patients or their relatives.

Eastman (1989), writing in the American Association of Retired Persons *News Bulletin*, stated tens of thousands of older people are living in an "inhuman and needless" stupor induced by misuse or overuse of prescription drugs. Eastman reported on an American Psychological Association (APA) forum which was held immediately after the release of a government report written by Richard P. Kusserow, Inspector General of the Department of Health and Human Services, about the widespread problem of mismedication among American's elderly.

"While overmedication calms or induces sleep in older patients and quiet, manageable patients lessen demands on nursing home staff, 'chemical restraints' could be deadly as well as unethical. Organic brain syndrome could be caused by drug intoxication helping to explain the report's findings that 51 percent of deaths from drug reactions involve people 60 years of age or older."

Government Involvement with Behavior Control

During the fifties and sixties, the Central Intelligence Agency (CIA) is known to have given drugs to prison inmates in Atlanta, Georgia, to determine changes in their behavior at various dosage levels.

- How much information was given to them about the possible long-term effects of these drugs?

Power of Suggestion

In a class assignment, students were asked to investigate the power of suggestion in advertisements on television. The students became very interested in their project once they discovered that suggestion is used in a number of ways to urge people to buy something.

The teacher arranged for the students to talk to her husband, who was in that line of work. He told them about subliminal advertisements.

He said that the mind can pick up something that is shown upside down, such as a statement that says "buy brand X," and that a message has to be flashed on the screen for only a fraction of a second for the mind to "see" and understand it.

Given the financial restraints in today's society and considering how important it is for teenagers to wear certain types of clothes to be accepted as part of the peer group, should advertisements for items used by teenagers be shown on television when they use subliminal messages? If not, why not? If so, what, if any, restrictions should be made for advertisers?

- Could any consent given by these prisoners be called "informed consent," as defined by the law and the American Medical Association (1986) in the Judicial Opinions?

The CIA admitted to giving LSD to some of its agents, using them as guinea pigs, as well as giving various mixtures of drugs to servicemen during the years 1959-73. Using people as living test tubes left residual emotional problems, and some of these veterans later produced children with unusual birth defects.

Hodierne (1979) interviewed Steve Bonner, a veteran, who was part of a 1967 drug experiment by the U.S. Army. After 10 years of emotional problems and the birth of his first child who was paralyzed from the waist down with an open spine and hydrocephalus, the Army had consented to send him documents detailing the 1967 drug experiment in which he participated. Similar questions are being asked by others among the 7,000 people the Army says took part in the experiments during the early days of the Cold War.

After being told the drugs were already in use and would have no long-term effects, Bonner gave his consent to test drugs that could be used to incapacitate enemy troops. His reactions were detailed in Hodierne's interview as "the most terrifying . . . experience I have ever had." No conclusions have been reached in this case. However, a 180 million dollar settlement has been made between the manufacturers of Agent Orange, a chemical defoliant, and Vietnam veterans. These veterans had multiple medical problems after being sprayed from the air with this compound which was absorbed through the skin.

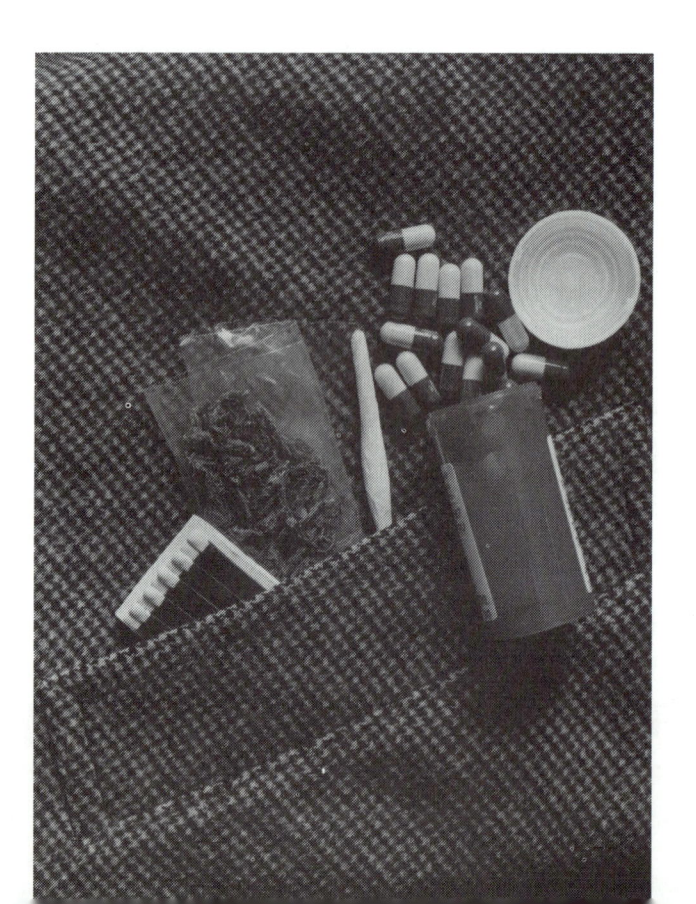

Alcohol and Recreational Drugs

National Center for Health Statistics data show alcohol was involved in three of the top causes of death in the United States in 1987. Motor vehicle accidents were fourth, suicide was eighth, and chronic liver disease and cirrhosis of the liver was ninth. Schoenberger (1987) reported that a survey of North Carolina students (grades 7-12) indicated that 60% of them had used alcohol and 40% had used marijuana.

Desmond (1987) wrote the cover story for *Time* titled, "Out in the Open," describing the 18 million Americans who have a drinking problem. With celebrities that include movie stars and First Ladies entering sanatoriums for treatment of alcoholism, the magnitude of this problem has started to unfold. According to Desmond:

"Alcoholism's toll is frightening. Cirrhosis of the liver kills at least 14,000 alcoholics a year. Drunk drivers were responsible for approximately half the 46,000 driving fatalities in the U.S. in 1986. Alcohol was implicated in up to 70% of the 4,000 drowning deaths last year and in about 30% of the nearly 30,000 suicides. A Department of Justice survey estimates that nearly a third of the nation's 523,000 state-prison inmates drank heavily before committing rapes, burglaries and assaults."

The government's "Be Smart" campaign (aimed at eight-to-twelve-year-olds), the Mothers Against Drunk Driving (MADD), and Students Against Drunk Driving (SADD) are trying to curb the use of alcohol with education and prevention. The effects of alcohol (which are very noticeable on social occasions) confirm that this indeed is a drug that modifies behavior. Alcohol is blamed for altering the behavior of the captain of the Exxon Valdez, causing what environmentalists call the country's worst disaster.

"'These are misdemeanors of such magnitude that have never been equaled in this country,' said New York Supreme Court Justice Kenneth Rohl as he sentenced the fired Captain of the Exxon Valdez for drunkenly grounding his oil-gorged tanker on a reef in Alaska's beautiful Prince William Sound," (Hackett, 1989).

Rosenblatt and Thomas (1986) call it "the enemy within." From harmless cure-alls in the late 19th century, cocaine and opium have become highly addictive drugs. Crack, so named because cocaine makes a cracking sound as it is boiled down, is the most addictive popular drug of all. With its devastating effects on the brain, there is no desire for food, sex, or sleep.

The cost to society can be enormous as bus drivers, train engineers, airplane pilots, and other public servants get hooked, and innocent consumers find themselves at risk. Headlines such as: "PCP involved in fatal wreck of Amtrak train" (1987) and "City police and firemen using illicit drugs" (Morganthau, 1986) are becoming too frequent. *Time, Newsweek,* and *Discover* have published more than a half dozen special reports on the rapid rise in drug abuse in America and the crime rate which rises along with it.

Drugs that alter the brain's biochemistry also assault the body and nervous system. Irritability, nervousness, sleeplessness, delusions, hallucinations, and other nightmares are never imagined by the user who seeks stimulation, euphoria, and perhaps sexual excitement. Seeking a thrill, drug users may pay for it with their lives.

Codes of Ethics

Whereas ancient philosophers made little distinction between legal obligation and ethical duty, the climate of the twentieth century is very different. Today, most legal requirements are minimal, while ethical or moral standards require the best performance we can deliver. We view ethics as beyond the province of law, calling us to actions that are nobler and more altruistic than those required by law. *The Hippocratic Oath* admonished physicians to "do no harm" to the patient. England's Sir Thomas Percival continued that idea when he wrote his book on medical ethics and was a strong influence on the English physicians who set sail on the Mayflower to come to the "new world" and begin medical practice. The American Medical Association, which was founded in 1847, drew up its own code of ethics which again asked physicians to "do no harm" to the patient. Over the next forty years, a rapidly changing society created new bioethical problems. The AMA responded to the needs of society by updating its Principles of Medical Ethics three times, while continuing to point out to the physician that he or she is responsible to the patient for as long as the therapy or its effects last.

The Geneva Convention Code of Medical Ethics was established by the World Medical Association in 1949; the Nuremberg Code was established because of World War II war crimes; and the Declaration of Helsinki was written to update worldwide guidelines on human experimentation. All these codes remind us of the sanctity of human life. When we stop to consider the full impact of tinkering with the life of a human being and the emerging issue of patients' rights, which has developed during the past ten to fifteen years, the ethical implications of controlling human behavior become more crucial (Chapman, 1984).

The President's Commission

Why do we have feelings of disquiet about the possibilities for evil as well as good in the matter of behavior control? In 1978, the United States Congress passed legislation establishing the President's Commission for the Study of Ethical Problems in Medicine and Biomedical and Behavioral Research, which was charged with investigating and reporting on key ethical issues in health care. One of the areas to be studied was human behavior controls relative to patient sovereignty. This Commission was to study social, legal, economic, and religious concerns involved in the important issues of bioethics. Some issues were conceptual in nature, but more of them related to conflicts over competing values. As Cook stated in a personal note at the conclusion of his novel, *Mindbend* (1985), medical ethics is losing ground to economic and business interests, and the American public has a right and an obligation to know what kind of system is evolving. Is the current watchword "let the buyer beware," instead of the historical, "do no harm to the patient?"

Summary

As new discoveries lead to profound ethical, social, and legal issues, we must rethink our ideas of personal responsibility. As we gain newer understanding of body chemistry, we begin to realize the enormous power for potential harm that we hold in controlling behavior of the human being. Let us consider forums for airing matters of concern. Perhaps we need to think of three new R's: re-examining, revising, and reaffirming our system of values and beliefs. The study of bioethics is timely and complex, with earth-shaping implications. Let us study the full implications of the emotionally wrenching decisions we often make in these situations and use our intelligence and our hearts to solve these new problems in health care delivery. The unthinkable will eventually meet the inevitable, and we must confront reality. If we are to create the kind of world we want to live in, we must consider what we are doing, make choices we can live with, and add to the body of wisdom we leave behind.

Cited References

Allman, W.F. (1989). Science 1, Advertisers 0. *U.S. News and World Report, 106,* (17), 60-61.

Andrews, L. (1977, March). Psychosurgery: the new Russian roulette. *New York,* 38-40.

Chapman, C.B. (1984). *Physicians, law and ethics.* New York: New York University Press.

Cook, R. (1983). *Brain.* New York: Putnam.

Cook, R. (1977). *Coma.* Boston: Little, Brown & Co.

Cook, R. (1985). *Mindbend.* New York, Putnam.

Cook, R. (1987). *Outbreak.* New York: Putnam.

Current Opinion of the Council on Ethical and Judicial Affairs of the American Medical Association. (1986). Illinois: AMA.

Desmond, E.W. (1987). Out in the open. *Time, 130* (22), 80-90.

Dillingham, S. (1987, September 14). Inaudible messages making a noise. *Insight,* 44-45.

Eastman, P. (1989). America's "other drug problem" overwhelms thousands. *AARP News Bulletin, 30* (4), pp. 1,3.

Garcia, G.X. (1988, July 10). Subliminal messages on Mexican TV. *Raleigh News and Observer.*

Goode, E.E. (1989). When mental illness hits home. *U.S. News and World Report, 106* (16), 55-65.

Grumman, C. (1987, November 17). Getting the message across. *Raleigh News and Observer.*

Hackett, G. (1989). Environmental politics. *Newsweek, 113* (16), 18-19.

Hodierne, R. (1979, October 22). Army drug experiments still haunt veteran. *The Charlotte Observer,* p. 1.

Key, W.B. (1973). *Subliminal seduction.* New Jersey: Prentice-Hall.

Lamar, Jr., J. V. (1986, The high price of abuse. *TIME, 127* (22), 16-18.

Many patients are drugged for ease of staff. (1989, March 13). *Raleigh Times* p. 4.

Morganthau, T. (1986, September 29). A question of privacy. *Newsweek,* 18-21.

PCP involved in fatal wreck of Amtrak train. (1987, March 26). *Raliegh News and Observer.*

President's Commission for the Study of Ethical Problems in Medicine and Biomedical and Behavioral Research. (1983). *Summing up.* Washington, D.C.: Government Printing Office.

Radio station runs subliminal messages to quit smoking habit. (1987, November 22). *Concord Tribune.*

Rosenblatt, R. and Thomas, E. (1986). Drugs: The enemy within. *TIME, 128* (11), 58-68.

Schoenberger, S. (1987, November 19). Teens using alcohol despite anti-drug efforts. *Raleigh News and Observer.*

Webster's Ninth New Collegiate Dictionary. (1984). Massachusetts: Merriam-Webster.

World Medical Association Handbook of Declarations. (1985). Farnborough, Hampshire: Inkon Printers.

Joe and the Cup of Coffee

Joe has been a teacher at Metropolitan High School for about fifteen years. He has been there longer than most of the teachers and a great deal longer than the principal. To a considerable extent, he does what he wants. During the last year or so he has taken to carrying his thermos of coffee wherever he goes. He teaches his classes with a coffee cup in one hand. Most of the students and some of the teachers know that the coffee is laced with whiskey.

A couple of the students get mad at Joe and write an anonymous note to the principal telling him about Joe's coffee cup. The principal asks to check the cup, saying he has heard it is not just plain coffee. Joe refuses. He claims this would be a violation of his right of privacy. Then the principal tells Joe that he can no longer bring his thermos to class. He is to purchase coffee from the vending machine just as the other teachers do. If he doesn't drink it during the break from class, he can take that into class with him. The principal says it is unprofessional to take the thermos to class with him.

Joe becomes very upset. Where he used to be relatively easygoing and would laugh and joke with the students, he now becomes abrupt. He loses his temper easily and gives the students difficult assignments to complete. He has nothing to do with the rest of the teachers. He also leaves the classroom early and is usually late to class. By the end of the first week without his thermos, few people like Joe.

Early Saturday morning Joe is picked up for drunken driving. It happens that the officer is a former student of Joe's and is concerned about him. However, Joe becomes very abusive and tries to hit the policeman. He also threatens to go home and get a gun and "fix" the officer if he doesn't let him go. As a result, Joe is restrained and taken to a nearby psychiatric hospital. Once there, he is given sedatives to control him. Joe continues to get the sedatives for some time but does not improve. Investigation shows that Joe has become addicted to the sedatives.

- Should a teacher who has a drinking problem but is doing a good job be dismissed or allowed to continue to work?

- Were the teachers who knew what was in Joe's cup wrong because they did not notify the principal about Joe's drinking?

- Were the students who wrote the anonymous note justified in reporting Joe?

- Should Joe have been allowed to continue teaching with his cup in the classroom?

- Should Joe be fired because he was picked up for driving while drunk?

- Should the principal or other teachers have noticed Joe's personality change? If so, did they have a responsibility to notify anyone?

- Would it be proper for the policeman to let Joe go home with a warning, rather than arrest him, because he knows Joe?

- Should Joe be allowed to return to his job after he is released from the hospital?

- Would you want Joe to teach a member of your family?

- If someone's actions do not cause harm to another individual, should the person be allowed to do as he or she pleases?

- Would society benefit if all people who acted in a way that could harm society were required to undergo human behavior control?

6

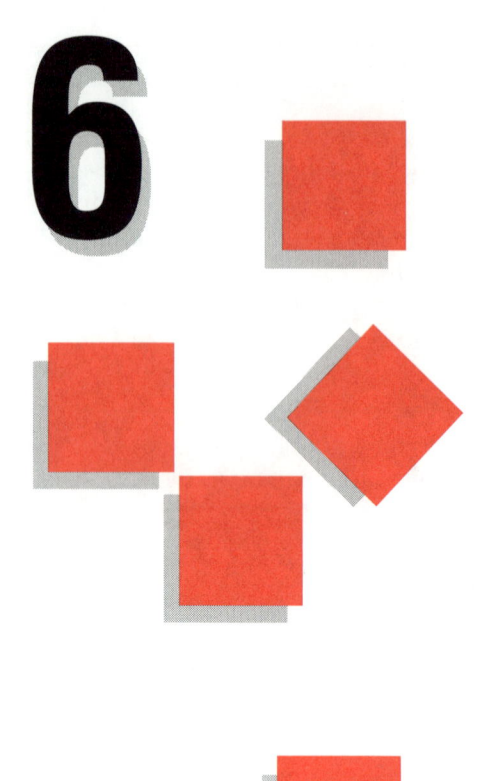

Fetal Research

Mildred M. Pittman*

Objectives

After reading this chapter you should be able to:

- Define the terms listed at the beginning of this chapter.
- State some rationales for in-utero invasion procedures.
- Discuss some generally accepted moral values associated with in-utero invasive procedures.
- Discuss some decision-making steps that might be involved in the interruption of a pregnancy.
- State some aspects of the controversy involving research conducted on fetal tissue ex-utero.

Terms and Definitions

Amniocentesis. Transabdominal puncture of the amniotic sac, using a needle and syringe, in order to remove amniotic fluid.
Fetal alcohol syndrome. Birth defects in infants born to mothers whose chronic alcoholism persisted during the gestation period.
Fetology. The study of fetuses.
Fetus. In humans, the child in-utero from the third month to birth; prior to that time it is called an embryo.
Alpha-fetoprotein. An antigen present in the human fetus; the amniotic fluid can be used to evaluate fetal development.
Ultrasonography. Use of ultrasound to produce an image or photograph of an organ or tissue, useful in fetology to determine gestational age, approximate weight, some anatomical malformations, and general condition.

Introduction

Research on the unborn, specifically the fetus, has gained prominence with the development of technology that permits assessment and diagnosis of imperfections. The technical advances and scientific discoveries have created specialization in **fetology.** In a broad interpretation, fetology involves not only physicians but geneticists, chemists, biologists, and other scientists.

Any research conducted on humans evokes moral, ethical, religious, and ultimately societal consideration. In addition, research conducted on fetuses commands particular consideration due to the dependency of the subjects and an absence of historical data. Why conduct research on fetuses? One response is so that we can accurately diagnose congenital anomalies such as neural tube defects (i.e., encephalocele, spina bifida, and meningocele). When diagnosis is not followed by interruption of the pregnancy, we must seek means to improve the quality of life for the infant so afflicted.

Having developed more accurate diagnoses, researchers now seek means of definitive treatment before birth as in the case of spina bifida. There is evidence that the trauma of birth maximizes the anomaly in many infants. This reaffirms the need to seek means of treatment before birth. Surgical procedures in-utero are classified as experimental due to the limited number of cases.

Other congenital anomalies have been treated by extrauterine surgery with a return to the womb for completion of the pregnancy. The treatment of other congenital anomalies including metabolic diseases, hormonal imbalance, blood dyscrasia, and specific fetal syndromes (for example, fetal alcohol syndrome) before birth is challenging. Less invasive, less traumatic means such as changes in the mother's diet have been documented as treatment as well.

Of course not all attempts to improve the quality of life for the child at birth are successful. All in-utero invasive procedures carry a high risk. All procedures/treatments involving fetuses result in a wide range of outcomes. Between the two extremes of overwhelming success and the death of the fetus occur a range of other outcomes. Any outcome less than overwhelmingly successful tends to evoke concern.

---

*Mildred M. Pittman
Unit Manager, Twin Lakes Hospital, Denton, Texas.

Ethical Issues: Preliminary Considerations

Let's look at some basics in ethics, specifically related to health and medical care. Smurl (1984) lists five moral values on which most people might agree even if they apply them differently "in the crunch."

These are:

1. Self-improvement or developing one's self through a coherent life plan.
2. Truth telling or communicating one's opinions accurately.
3. Promise keeping or doing what you agreed to.
4. Beneficence or doing what is in another's best interest, or at least not harming another.
5. Justice or acting fairly in our exchanges with others and, insofar as we have control over resources, in the way we allocate the benefits and burdens of these resources.

Of these, beneficence is most often listed as relevant to fetal research.

- Is ethics the same thing as morality?
- Is morality the same as mores/customs or perhaps the same as a law?

Smurl provides definitions that show us the differences:

- **Customs** are traditional ways of doing things, and they give rise to group rules claiming we are obliged to continue them.
- **Laws** are standards of conduct promulgated by legitimate authorities and are enforced by the police powers of governments.
- A **morality** is a fairly well-organized set of judgments about what's right and wrong for humans generally.
- **Ethics** is the organized study of the foundations for and the applications of moralities.

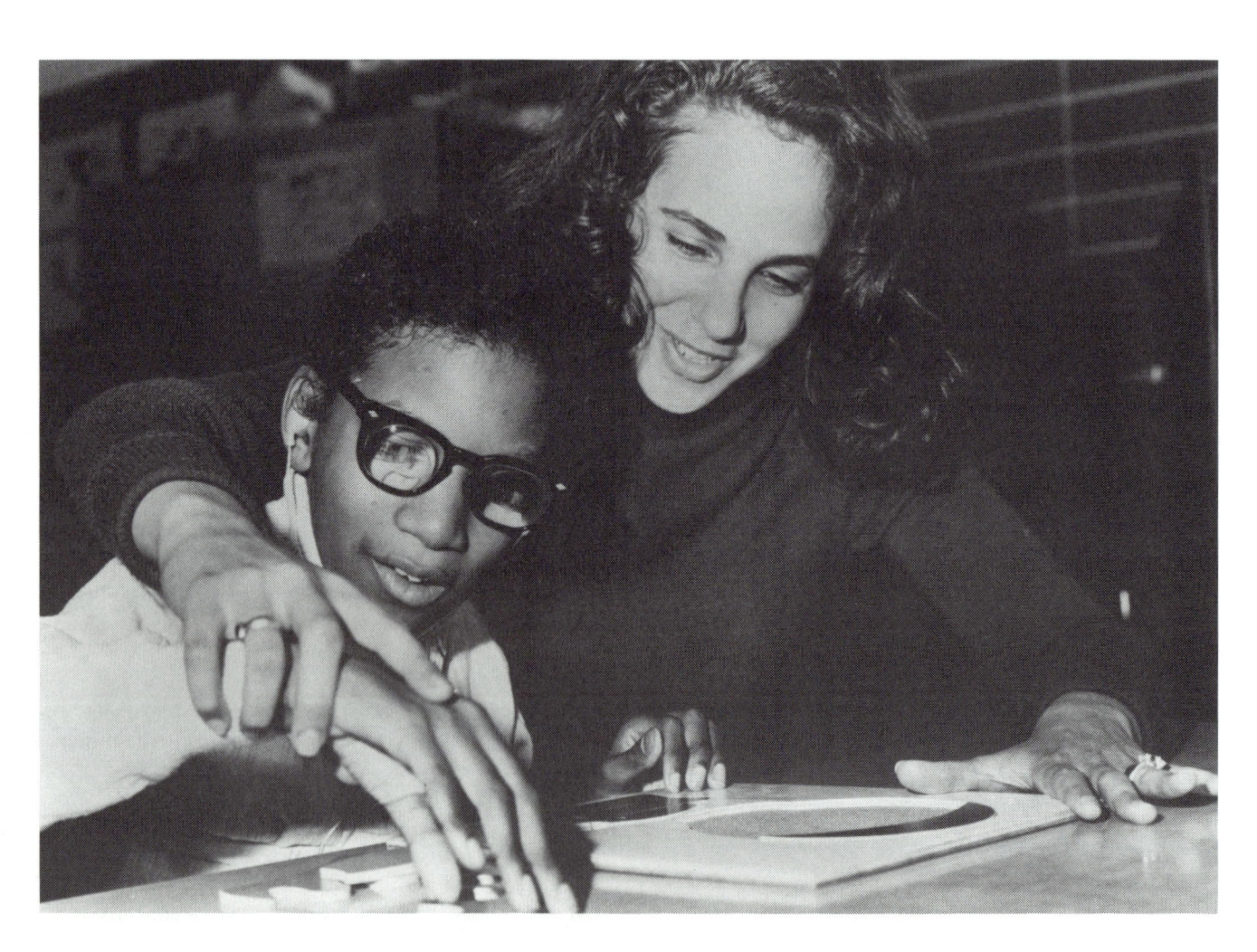

When faced with hard moral choices, how do people decide and then account for what they think is morally right? Smurl explains that moral dilemmas are hard choices between two perfectly good values or between honoring two quite reasonable moral rules or principles. The dilemma occurs because we are unable to respect both equally and must give priority to one. If people do not evade these decisions, pass them off to others, or refuse to explain their choices, then they usually tend to resolve moral dilemmas on one or more of the following levels.

"Gut" Level Approach

This approach works well enough to resolve dilemmas, but people find it hard to explain the reasons for their choices. Decisions made on this level can be quite satisfactory if the problem is a customary one and if the person is habitually honest and accountable. Otherwise, and especially if they aim to explain the reasons for their choices, they usually move to one or more of the next three levels of decision making.

Level of Rules

The moral, legal, and professional level of rules approach is populated with very specific and highly directive "do's" and "don'ts." Rules act as guides for decisions and can be appealed to as reasons for choices. Rules can conflict, however, and because they are so specific they can justify either a "do" or "don't do" decision. When the rules conflict, choices must be made on one or both of the next two levels of moral reasoning and discourse.

Level of Principles

Moral principles are composed of more general, commonly human, and impartial guidelines. Some of these principles are stated positively, setting out goals and directions. Others are stated negatively, setting down limits or boundaries and are often considered to be more stringent. They offer no panaceas in moral dilemmas, however, because they can be misstated or poorly applied. They can also be unsystematic and mutually contradictory and, in the case of really hard choices, they almost always require some sort of ranking. Thus, in attempts to explain their principles, the basis for them, and the priority they assign to one or more, people often need to appeal to the next level of discourse.

Level of Premises

The level of premises represents the bases and grounds of decisions, one's loyalties and commitments, goals and desires, and the central beliefs, stories, and other "master interpretations" of meaning and value which people consider true, good, and beautiful. These premises are often and necessarily nonrational but not necessarily antirational. They can be explained and defended, but they more commonly function as nonrational sources of self-respect or respect for other.

Among premises are some which suggest the best way to decide. When making and explaining hard moral choices, people appeal to several reasonable methods of decision making. The three most common are:

1. **Duty-based approaches** which make the decision turn on a judgment that an action fulfills an obligation or that it would fail to do what's owed others.
2. **Results-based approaches** which make the decision turn on a calculation of results achievable.
3. **Rights-based approaches** which make the decision turn on the answer to the questions whether or not there is a valid claim to something or a valid claim to be able to do something or a claim that others should refrain from doing something to you.

None of these approaches excludes considerations from the other categories. What distinguishes them is what they make decisive, the "bottom line" on which they make the decision turn. For example, when using the duty-based approach, rights and results are often important considerations but they will not be as decisive as are considerations of duty.

This review of ethics quickly demonstrates the many societal forces that contribute to individual decisions related to fetal research.

Responsive Decision Making

The findings in genetic screening often require quick decisions. Fortunately, for many, the findings substantiate the expectation of a healthy well-developed newborn. However, when the findings suggest the high probability of a congenital anomaly, there may be a strong recommendation for interruption of the pregnancy. When the findings are inconclusive, there may well be indecisiveness regarding whether to interrupt or continue the pregnancy.

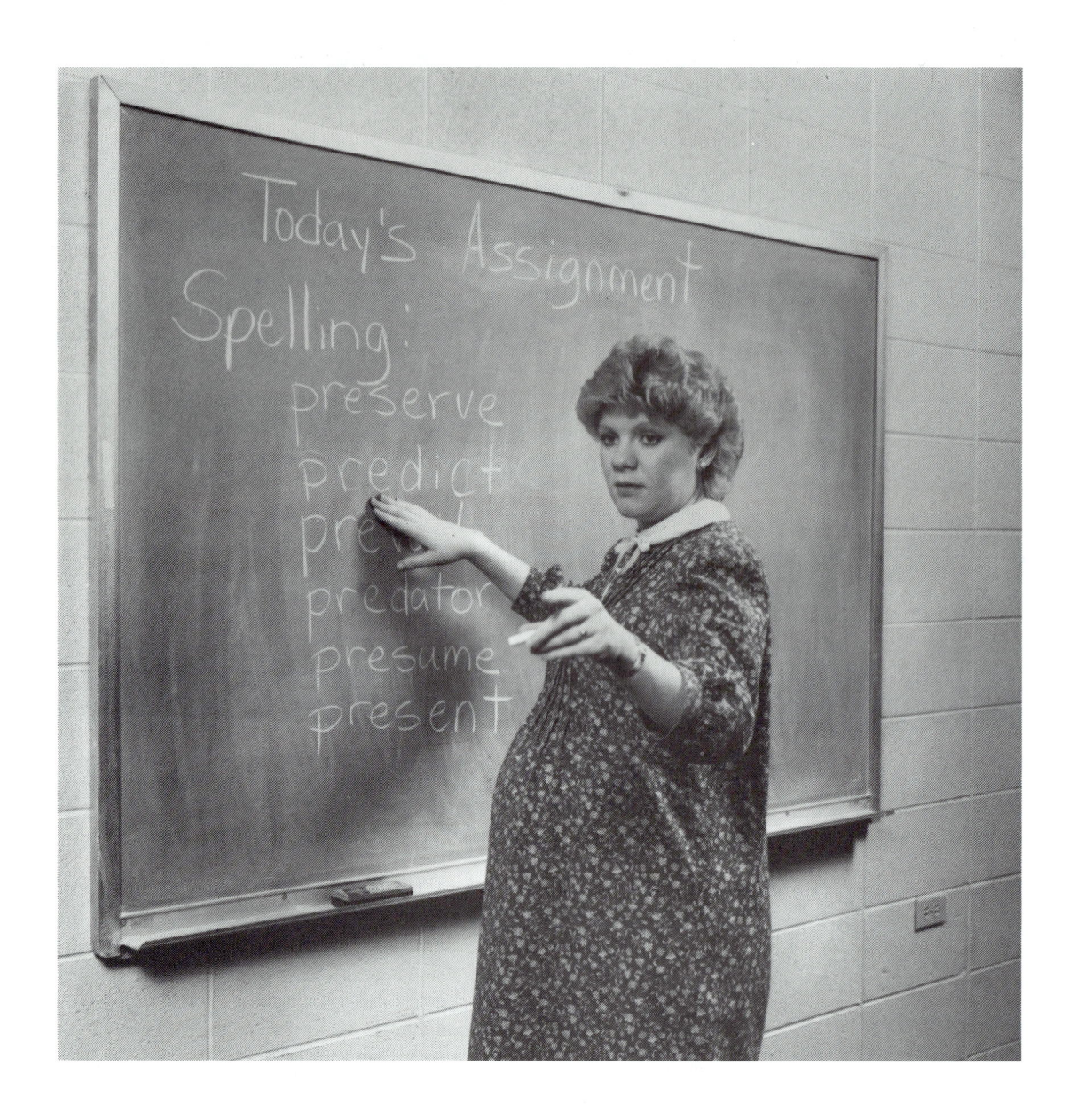

An Experimental Operation

Louisa and Michael have been married for about six years. They have four children, and Louisa is three months pregnant. A week ago Michael lost his job.

Louisa has not been feeling well so when she goes to the clinic today with the children, she asks the doctor to look at her also. He does so and tells her that the baby has a problem, but, as he is conducting research on this condition, he will operate on the fetus and follow its course without charge. The other option involves an abortion because of the effect of the problem on the fetus.

What should Louisa and Michael do?

The pregnant woman's informed consent is paramount to any decision to interrupt as is her implied consent to the continuance of the pregnancy. In the same manner, the treatment of any fetus, either by invasive or noninvasive means in-utero is contingent upon consent to do so. Most circumstances require both parents' agreement.

The circumstances in which the mother is declared incompetent or otherwise legally determined "unfit" has precedence. The declaration of "unfit" due to the mental/physical condition as a basis for interruption of the pregnancy is infrequent but garners vivid description in lay publications such as public newspapers. When medical records are pursued, they reveal specific cases and the criteria considered when declaring the mother "unfit."

In addition, institutions have established panels or committees which either determine the policies and/or review the reported cases. The committees usually have persons other than physicians as members. These groups then provide input from various disciplines and give the individual the benefit of their diverse backgrounds.

When seeking informed consent, the researcher must provide information about the procedures, risk, expected outcomes, costs, and any other related inquiry that the mother or parents make. Given the information, the mother or parents then make a decision. Such decisions are made by various means. Many such decisions are not predictable.

Many fetal procedures are still considered research and not standard medical practice. Fetal blood sampling can yield information for karyotyping and perhaps correcting malformations (Farah et al., 1986; Oliver and Ager, 1988). Intrauterine transfusion for rhesus disease is successful (Nicolaides et al., 1986). The insertion of a prosthesis to decrease intracranial pressure in a hydrocephalic fetus by creating a shunt diversion also has been successful (Clewell et al., 1986).

Some neural tube defects have been closed by in-utero surgery, and Chervenak (1988) had success with the management of fetal teratomas. This list is not inclusive and is being expanded. An international registry has been established to record experimental surgical interventions (Fetal Therapy, 1988) so that accurate records can be maintained and adequate counseling offered to parents of unborn children with congenital defects.

Even more dramatic procedures have been described; for example, obstructive uropathy is the most common type of anomaly treated by urinary tract surgery (Farah et al., 1986). In some circumstances, a hysterotomy is performed; the baby is operated on and returned to the uterus to develop until term (Manning, 1986).

Research Using Fetal Tissue

Additional consideration must be given to research conducted on fetal tissue ex-utero. The expelled fetus is not classified as alive for a lengthy interval as separation of the placenta from the uterine wall deprives the fetus of all nutrients. The entire aborted fetus must be disposed of according to existing state and national regulation.

Research using a portion of an expelled fetus (fetal tissue) must comply with existing institutional policy developed in accordance with these regulations. "Current federal regulations permit the use of tissue from dead fetuses in experimental transplantations when it is conducted in accordance with state law," (Annas, 1985). A twenty-one member Human Tissue Fetal Transplant Research Panel, created by the National Institutes of Health (NIH), concluded that "although it was of 'moral relevance' that the fetal tissue be obtained from an induced abortion (rather than a spontaneous abortion or an interrupted ectopic pregnancy), the use of the tissue in research was 'acceptable public policy' because 'abortion is legal and . . . the research in question is intended to achieve significant medical goals."

Summary

Ethical dilemmas are not new, only the circumstances are new. The past serves as a guide to the present and influences the future. Unfortunately, decisions regarding fetal research, specifically in-utero treatment, most often must be made with little time delay. The later stages of development may provide relatively conclusive evidence of an anomaly, but a disadvantage is that a decision to abort or to treat or not treat in-utero must be made almost immediately.

The effects of the decision extend for at least a lifetime and sometimes two generations. Health care providers must accept the challenge these ethical dilemmas present. The concept of providing individuals with many resources from which to make a decision constitutes the informed consent principle. This principle will play a major role in ultimately determining the ethics of fetal research.

Cited References

Annas, George J. (1985, March). Letter: embryo research. *The Lancet*, 1: 8427: 522.

Chervenak, Frank A., M.D. and Larber, John, M.D. (1988). *Anomalies of the fetal head, neck, and spine: ultrasound diagnosis and management*. Philadelphia: Saunders.

Clewell, William H., M.D.; Manco-Johnson, Michael L., M.D.; and Manchester, David K., M.D. (1986, September). Diagnosis and management of fetal hydrocephalus. *Clinical Obstetrics and Gynecology*, 29: 3: 514-22.

Farah, Solange B., Ph.D.; Simpson, Thomas J., M.D.; and Gollus, Mitchell S., M.D. (1986, September). Hematopoietic stem cells for the treatment of genetic disease. *Clinical Obstetrics and Gynecology*, 29: 3: 543-50.

Fetal therapy: ethical considerations. American Academy of Pediatrics Committee of Bioethics. (1988, June). *Pediatrics,* 81: 6: 898,899.

Greely, T. et al. (1989, April 20). Special report: the ethical use of human fetal tissue in medicine. *The New England Journal of Medicine*, 320: 16: 1079-82.

Manning, Frank A., M.D. (1986, September). International fetal surgery registry: 1985 update. *Clinical Obstetrics and Gynecology,* 29: 3: 551-57.

Nicolaides, K. H., Todeck, C. H., Soothill, P. W., and Campbell, S. (1986, May 10). Ultrasound guided sampling of umbilical cord placental blood to assess fetal well-being. *The Lancet*, 1: 1065-67.

Oliver, R. W. A., and Ager, R. P. (1988, March 26). Screening for Down's syndrome. *The Lancet*, 1: 8587: 709-10.

Smurl, F. (1984) *A Primer in Ethics*. Indiana University, Indianapolis.

The Artificial Placenta

The shortage of children available for adoption is well documented. Recognizing that there needs to be some means of making more children available for adoption, a researcher decides to investigate developing an artificial placenta to replace the human one.

He works for the next three years and finally is successful. He develops an artificial placenta that will sustain fetal life. Wanting to share this good news with others, he writes a paper to tell the scientific community about his research. He indicates that by placing test tube embryos in the artificial placenta, a child can be brought to term. He goes on to say that he believes that by using this method anyone who wants a child will be able to have one to care for and love. He offers to provide a few people with a child within a year. He does say, however, that he must charge a sizeable fee for the service in order to recover the money he spent in conducting the research.

- What about the embryos that do not "make it" in the artificial placenta?

- What about the people who can't afford to pay the fee for such a child?

- Does the scientist have the right to try to retrieve the money he spent in his research?

- What obligation does the researcher have to parents and the child?

- Do people volunteering the sperm or egg have a right to say what will happen to it?

- Suppose there is an abnormality later in life. Who should be responsible for the financial care of the child?

- Regarding a baby resulting from this technique, what obligation do the parents have to continue reporting information about the baby's development?

- Who should establish the criteria for the male and female biological parents?

- What effect might this have on the family structure?

- Would you feel as though you had a baby if it were "grown" in a laboratory?

- Is this method any different from using the services of a surrogate mother? If so, how?

- What moral and ethical responsibilities does a world power country have regarding this type of research?

7

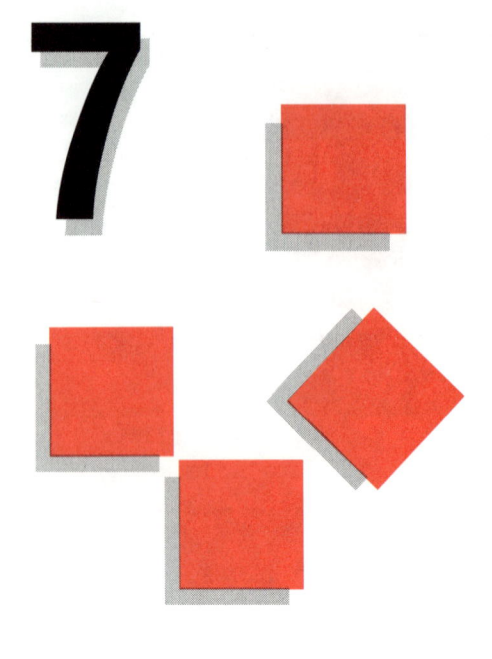

Mass Screening for Genetic Disorders

Mildred M. Pittman*

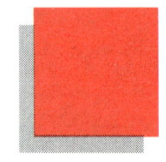

Objectives

After reading this chapter, you should be able to:

- Define the terms listed at the beginning of this chapter.
- List four major genetic screening populations.
- List two common diseases for which carriers can be detected by genetic screening.
- Describe potential patterns for genetic screening.

Terms and Definitions

Amniocentesis. Transabdominal puncture of the amniotic sac using a needle and syringe to remove amniotic fluid.

Autosomal recessive. Circumstance in which both parents of an affected child appear essentially normal, but, by chance, both carry the same harmful gene although neither may be aware of it.

Chromosome. A structure in the nucleus of a cell containing a linear thread of DNA, which transmits genetic information.

Fetoscopy. Examination of the fetus.

Genetic screening. A systematic search in a population for persons of certain genotypes.

Genotypes. Basic combination of genes of an organism.

Heterozygote. An individual with different alleles for a given characteristic (one or two or more different genes containing specific inheritable characteristics that occupy corresponding positions on paired chromosomes.)

Polymorphism. Capacity for appearing in many forms, existence of several types in the same group or species.

X-linked recessive. Normal females have two X chromosomes; normal males have one X and one Y; usually, a clinically normal mother carries a faulty gene on one of her X chromosomes.

Introduction

Screening for genetic disorders is an outstanding demonstration of effective scientific cooperation utilizing high technology in an attempt to aid society in solving a series of persistent human imperfections.

Genetic screening can be viewed as an organized or systematic search for persons of a certain genetic makeup **(genotypes)** in a selected population. It can also refer to identification of an unrecognized disease or defect in an apparently healthy individual.

Mass screening of the general population obviously would help identify carriers, but it also presents many problems and questions:

- Who gets screened and why?
- Who pays for the screening?
- Who has access to the results?
- What use is made of the results?

In this chapter, we will look at some of these issues and will present a basis for understanding what genetic screening entails. A limited amount of screening is already being done, but current research efforts will increase the amount of screening possible. Let's first look at the goals of screening programs.

Genetic Screening

Genetic screening is a search in a population for:

- persons who possess genotypes that are associated with the development of genetic diseases.
- persons with certain genotypes that are known to predispose the individual to illness.
- persons who are the **heterozygous** carriers of recessively inherited genes that in **autosomal recessive** disorders (double dose) can cause genetic disease in their descendants.
- persons with **polymorphisms** (variations) not now known to be associated with a disease state.

National Academy of Sciences
Committee for the Study of

Inborn Errors of Metabolism

---

*Mildred M. Pittman
Unit Manager, Twin Lakes Hospital, Denton, Texas.

Purpose and Goals

Some of the goals of genetic screening are:

Medical interventions – depending on the severity of the defect (condition), physicians may advise termination of a pregnancy, alternative conception modes, and/or sterilization.

Reproductive information and choices – this information would provide realistic and reasonable alternatives to the typical conceptual pattern including artificial insemination, selective termination of a pregnancy in which a fetus has a proven defect, sterilization, and adoption, among others.

Prenatal diagnosis – identification of fetal defects, i.e., before birth. These diagnoses are determined by fetoscopy, fetography, amniocentesis, and other procedures.

Identification of susceptibility to disease – historical information regarding susceptibility of populations provides a basis for genetic research of select individuals.

Research and education – identification of carrier suspects must be determined by scientific means. In addition, the ultimate goal is more information on which couples can make decisions about parenting.

Treatment – medical, surgical, or psychiatric management will be dependent upon the severity of the problem and the wishes of the family, particularly parents.

Supportive management – early diagnosis of fetal conditions usually apparent only at birth will provide an opportunity to aid parents in decision making; this must be supportive in nature.

Genetic counseling – advising a family on the human problems that may arise from the occurrence or risk of occurrence of a genetic disorder in a family.

Basically, screening provides information from which individuals can make more informed decisions regarding genetic related health care needs.

ESTIMATED AVERAGE ANNUAL NUMBER OF LIVE BIRTHS WITH SPECIFIED BIRTH DEFECTS, UNITED STATES, 1970-1979

Clubfoot	9000
Rh Disease of the Newborn	8800
Hip Dislocation	7100
Cleft Palate and/or Cleft Lip	5000
Open Spine and/or Water on the Brain	2900
Down syndrome	2800
Webbed Fingers and/or Toes	2000
Cystic Fibrosis	200

Source: Center for Disease Control
(These estimates are based on hospital discharge notices covering about one third of the births in the United States. Only those structural defects evident at birth are shown.)

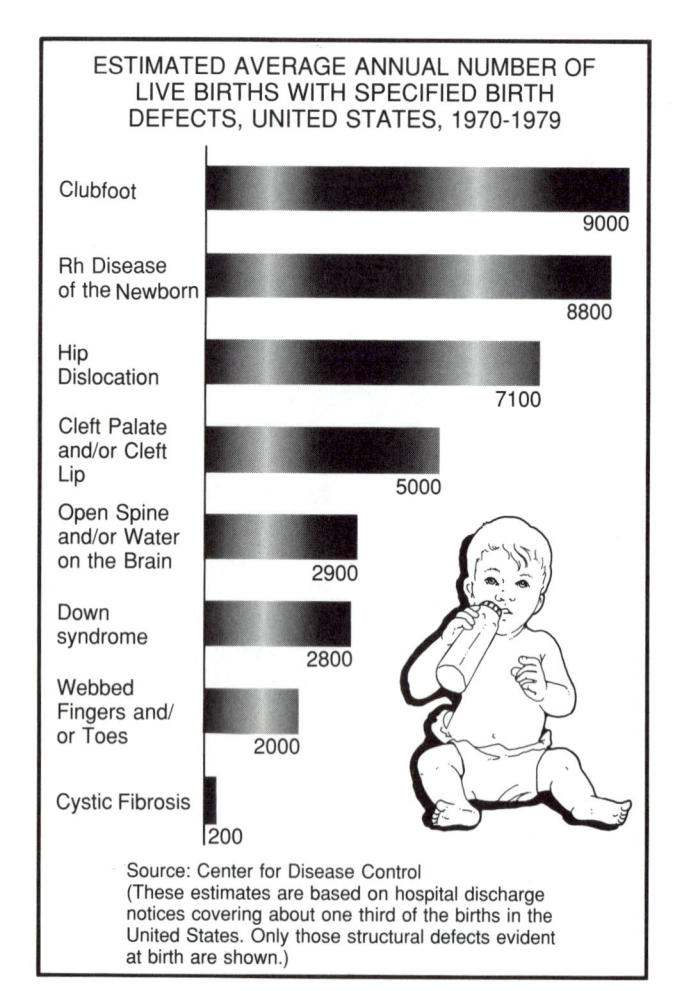

Estimated average annual number of live births with specified birth defects in the United States, 1970-1979.

Populations Undergoing Genetic Screening

The majority of all genetic screening is completed during the prenatal and neonatal life spans. Both men and women in the reproductive age groups constitute the next largest group. However, screening of individuals in the workplace is gaining emphasis.

Program Planning

Genetic screening programs of any group or groups require considerable planning and, of course, justification. The detection of disease in most circumstances compels that the diseased individual receive primary consideration. However, detection of genetic disease includes a broader scope of humanity, including future generations. This potential involvement of large segments of the population demands consideration of the following:

* **The importance of the disease.** While any disease is important to the individual or individuals afflicted, screening processes must be utilized when either large numbers are affected (directly or indirectly) or a select population has been identified as high risk.

* **The availability of screening test or tests.** This consideration appears self-apparent. Since the need for accuracy is critical, screening should not be done with tests that are unreliable or inconsistently reliable.

* **The natural history of the disorder in question.** Is there any advantage in making a diagnosis before symptoms appear? Can a latent period be determined? Is there a particular treatment that can alter the disease pattern?

* **The appropriateness and feasibility of screening procedures.** Any screening procedures should have clear goals, as well as facilities and personnel to provide appropriate education of the lay and professional segments of the target population. There must also be adequate diagnostic referral, follow up, and counseling services with comprehensive record keeping.

* **Cost-benefit and cost-effectiveness.** Current budget constraints in the entire health care delivery system demand careful scrutiny of costs. Preventing mental retardation by early dietary intervention, as is the case with hypothyroidism, and avoiding the resultant institutional cost burden give a clear example of cost-effectiveness. Another economically sound practice is to use screening procedures that can serve to verify the presence or absence of more than one defect at a time (Cohen, 1984).

Screening to Detect Carriers

Cohen (1984, p. 159) declares that "each person is a carrier for 5-7 recessive harmful genes for rare disorders." The purpose of carrier screening is the identification of heterozygotes for autosomal recessive or X-linked recessive disease.

Most carriers are healthy and recognized only with the delivery of an affected infant; however, the recognition of a heterozygous state before conception may allow the best chance for prevention of defects in infants. The two conditions most commonly screened for are Tay-Sachs disease and sickle-cell anemia.

Tay-Sachs Disease

Tay-Sachs disease is one of the most tragic inherited conditions. It first appears in its victims at the age of six months. An apparently healthy baby stops smiling, crawling, and turning over, loses its ability to grasp or reach out, and gradually becomes blind, paralyzed, and unaware of the surrounding world. Death occurs usually by the age of 3-4 years.

Screening for these carriers has been labeled "prototype" since this is the first disorder for which large-scale carrier screening was done in the United States. Perhaps one reason is the identification of a high-risk population, in this case, Jews of Eastern European ancestry, particularly from one area of Poland and Lithuania. However, more credit is due to the education

---

Chromosome Defects

A major medical center obtains a research grant to screen all newborn children in the city for chromosomal defects. In the course of conducting the screening, they locate a male infant who has an XYY chromosome structure. (Research indicates that individuals who have this chromosome structure tend to have antisocial tendencies. Indeed, many studies show that many criminals have an XYY structure.)

This infant is scheduled for adoption. Should the prospective parents be informed?

of both the religious and medical communities, which was not begun until technical aspects of the program were fully developed. Screening was begun in 1972 in communities near Baltimore and Washington. Some researchers estimate that only 10 percent of the population was tested.

Sickle-Cell Anemia

Sickle cell disease is an anemia primarily of the red blood cells in which these cells are misshapen so they resemble sickles and are less able to transport sufficient oxygen. The disease manifests itself as anemia and further results in "sickle cell crisis" which can be life threatening if not treated adequately.

Detection of the carriers of sickle-cell trait is a significant undertaking. In this circumstance, the high-risk population is the black race, with individuals of Mediterranean ancestry also showing a higher frequency of sickle-cell than other population groups. Screening began in the early 1970s, and now approximately 7-9 percent of black Americans are thought to have the sickle-cell trait. While the disease can be diagnosed in newborns, screening to identify carriers is important in genetic counseling. If it was revealed that you carried the sickle-cell trait, would you start a family or not?

Screening of Newborns

Phenylketonuria (PKU) is a disease that affects the way the body is able to process the food it takes in. Children born with PKU cannot metabolize a part of the protein phenylalanine, which then collects in the bloodstream. This abnormal buildup of phenylalanine can prevent the brain from developing as it should.

Initially, newborn screening programs were instituted for the detection of **phenylketonuria (PKU)**. Currently, more than twenty genetic and metabolic disorders can be screened for in the neonatal period, and that number is expanding (Cohen, 1984). Among those currently being tested for are the following:

- **Inborn errors of metabolism**, i.e., inherited biochemical defects, which include both enzyme deficiency and disease caused by enzyme product accumulation or enzyme product deficiency.
- **Phenylketonuria (PKU)** constitutes a major success story in newborn screening. Begun in 1961 it is now rare to see a child manifest the full spectrum of symptoms resulting from classic PKU. In fact, women who were diagnosed with PKU as infants are now having children. Inheritance is by the autosomal recessive mode of transmission for all but one variant (VI) which appears to be X-linked recessive.
- **Hypothyroidism.** The inclusion of this condition in neonatal screening is described as a "significant advance" in the prevention of mental retardation (Cohen, 1984, p. 165). Since some estimates indicate that 1-2 percent of the mentally retarded admitted to institutions may be hypothyroid, it is easy to see the societal effect of early diagnosis and prompt treatment.

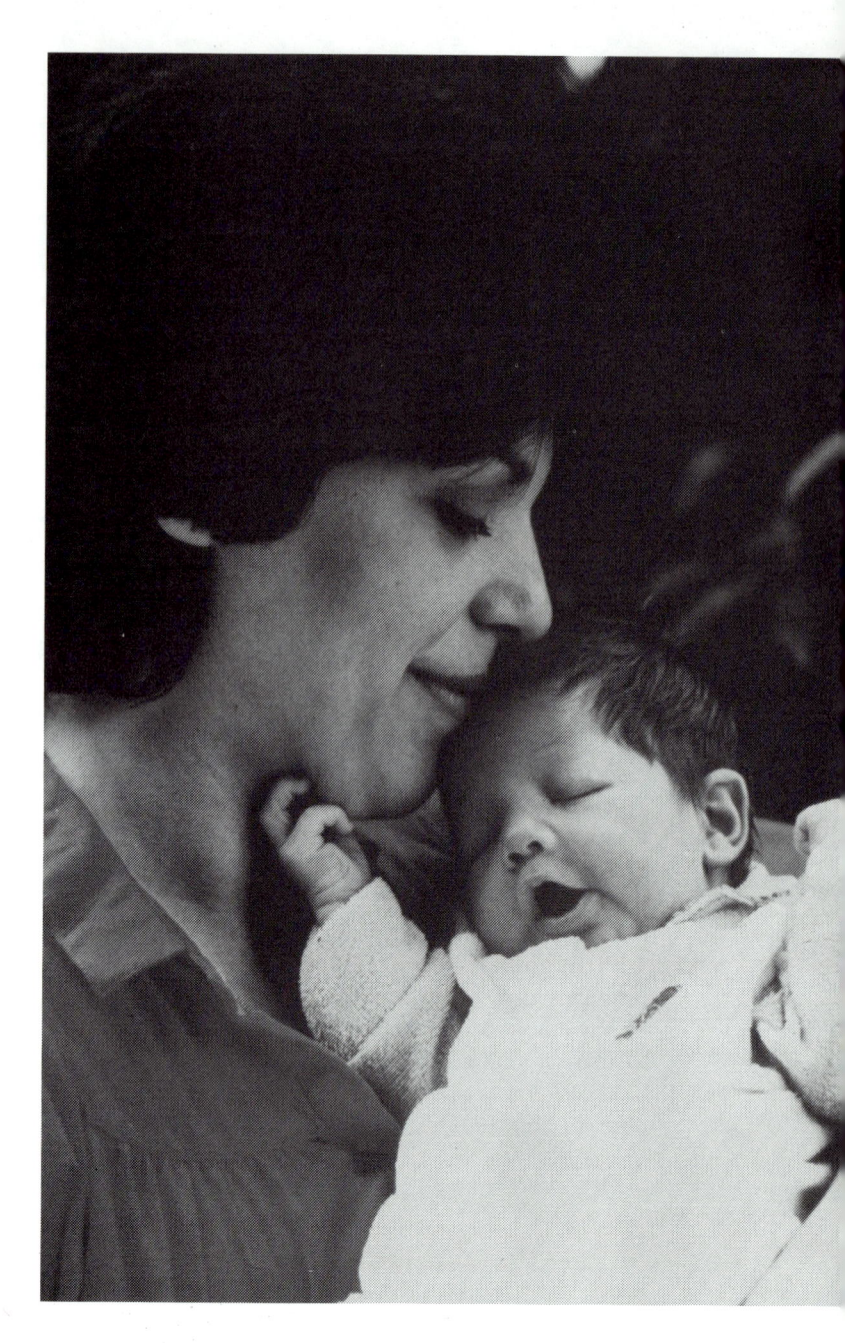

- **Metabolic disorders,** i.e., **tyrosinemia** (autosomal recessive), with an estimated occurrence in 1 of 50,000-100,000 births; **galactosemia** (autosomal recessive), in 1 of 50,000 births; **homocystinuria** (autosomal recessive), in 1 of 100,000-300,000 births, although a high-risk population is identified in Iceland; **maple-syrup urine disease (MSUD)** (autosomal recessive), in 1 of 180,000-225,000 births, although the incidence for Amish from Pennsylvania may be 1 of only 176 births; **histidinemia** (probably autosomal recessive), in 1 of 15,000 births and included primarily for research purposes; and **Hartnup disease** (not verified as autosomal recessive), in 1 of 16,000 live births nationwide.

- **Adenosine deaminase deficiency (ADA)** is currently included in the screening of newborns in New York. This disease is transmitted in the autosomal recessive pattern, and estimates of the occurrence in live births can only be projected.

- **Cystic fibrosis, Duchenne muscular dystrophy,** and **tuberous sclerosis,** plus others have been the subject of intensive research to facilitate the early – and, it is hoped, more effective – management of the disease entity.

Screening of newborns is not easily achieved. Modern care of newborns has shortened the hospital stay to hours rather than days, and some abnormalities cannot be accurately detected at such an early age. Follow-through after the infants have been discharged often is erratic and unreliable. Mass newborn screening (particularly in low-risk populations) is considered an unnecessary expense by states, which are now scrutinizing program cuts.

What Do States Screen For?

Cystic fibrosis – an inherited disease, present at birth, which causes certain glands to malfunction.

Duchenne muscular dystrophy – a disease marked by wasting and progressive weakness of skeletal muscles. This disease usually begins in the large muscles of lower trunk and upper legs.

Galactoseminia – condition marked by an inadequate amount of galactose, an enzyme or proteolytic ferment of milk.

Hartnup disease – a rare hereditary metabolic disease where amino acid absorption and excretion are abnormal, especially that of tryptophan.

Histidinemia – an inherited disease characterized by insufficient amount of the enzyme histidase which acts on 1-histidine.

Homocystinuria – an inherited disease caused by the absence of the enzyme essential to the metabolism of homocystine.

Maple-syrup urine disease – an inherited metabolic disease so named because of the characteristic odor of the urine and sweat. Clinically, in the first few months of life, there is a rapid deterioration of the nervous system and then death at an early age.

Tuberous sclerosis – a syndrome manifested by convulsive seizures, progressive mental disorder, adenoma sebacum, and tumors of the kidneys and brain with projections into the cerebral ventricles.

Tyrosinemia – a condition marked by inadequate amounts of tyrosinase, an enzyme which acts on tyrosine to produce melanin.

Screening Donors for Artificial Insemination

Artificial insemination is an option for persons who are known carriers of an undesirable autosomal recessive gene or for males who are affected by (or at risk for carrying) an autosomal dominant or X-linked mutant gene. When considering donors, every effort should be taken to exclude those individuals at greater risk than the general population. Possible indications for exclusion include:

- single gene disorder
- chromosome abnormality
- a hereditary disorder resulting from the combined action of several factors in the individual or close blood relatives
- Rh or ABO blood group that might cause incompatibility
- age of individual is forty-five years or older
- exposure to drugs, radiation, or chemical mutagens

- unexplained stillbirths, multiple miscarriages, or fetal deaths in the individual's own children or close blood relatives
- congenital hypothyroidism, a condition at birth where the thyroid hormone produced by the body is less than normal

Fetal Screening

Since 90 percent of the infants with neural tube defects (NTDs) are born to mothers with no prior history or known risk, screening for NTDs sounds appropriate.

NTDs are some of the most serious abnormalities of the central nervous system. They include absence of all or part of the brain, failure of the spinal column to close, and other malformations of the brain.

NTDs can now be detected by **amniocentesis** and **ultrasound**. Amniocentesis involves the examination of fluid withdrawn from the amniotic sac. The fetal protein, alpha-fetoprotein, is elevated in the amniotic fluid of more than ninety percent of the fetuses with open neural tube defects. So examining the amniotic fluid for this chemical is a good way to detect this type of defect.

However, amniocentesis does carry some risk. Also, the expense and drain on resources would be too great to make it useful in mass screening of low-risk persons. NTDs occur in 1.5 per 1000 live births.

Ultrasound techniques currently are not precise enough for use alone as a screening procedure. This technique is continually being refined and improved and may be a valuable method in the future.

What is the distinction between **fetal screening** and **prenatal diagnosis**? If screening is interpreted as a procedure completed on everyone, in this case pregnant women, the term is probably inaccurate. In the United States not all pregnant women are screened for genetic disorders. If, however, the term **screening** is used in a context of checking large numbers of persons to verify the presence or absence of a genetic disorder, its use may be more appropriate than diagnosis. Contemporary dictionaries define **diagnosis** as the act or process of identifying or determining the nature of a disease through examination.

Amniocentesis: When Should It Be Done?

The most common recommendations for amniocentesis include:

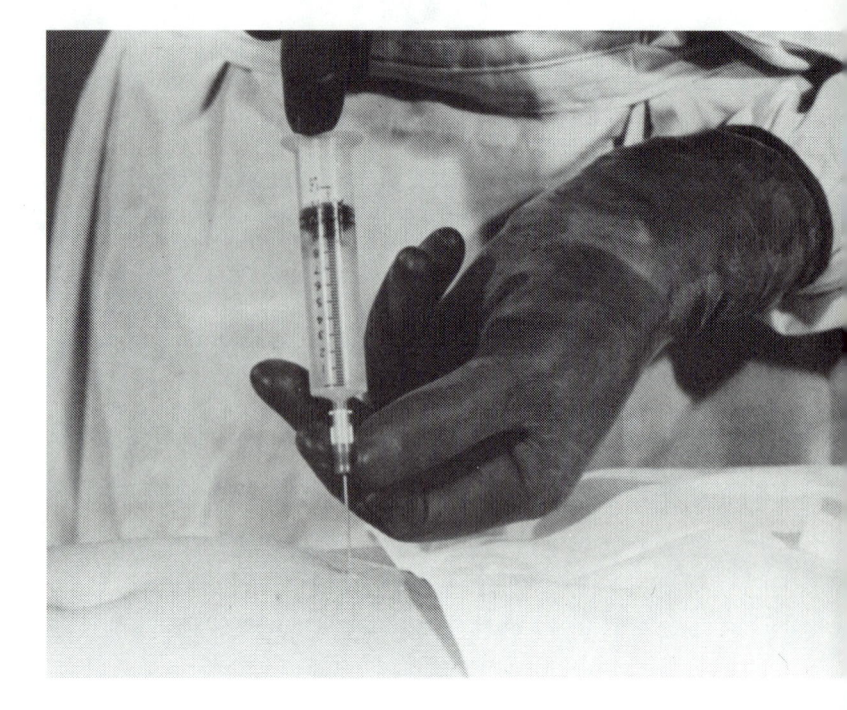

- Pregnancy at risk for chromosome aberration, including such factors as maternal age of thirty-five and over and a previous child with chromosome abnormality or instability disorder.
- Pregnancy at risk for NTDs, including high maternal serum level of alpha-fetoprotein and a previous child with NTDs.
- Pregnancy at risk for X-linked inherited disorders, as when the mother is a known carrier or when a close male relative of the mother is affected.
- Pregnancy at risk for detectable inherited biochemical disorder when parents are known carriers or when a previous child was born with known detectable biochemical disorder.
- Other circumstances, such as when there is a high degree of parental anxiety; when there has been significant environmental exposure to radiation, chemicals or drugs; or when the mother is diabetic.

Ultrasound: A Variety of Uses

Although used routinely in early pregnancy screening in Great Britain, ultrasound is not employed as routinely in the United States. However, ultrasound is the imaging method of first choice. Ultrasound imaging can begin around the fifth week. Fetal development can then be followed until delivery, if necessary.

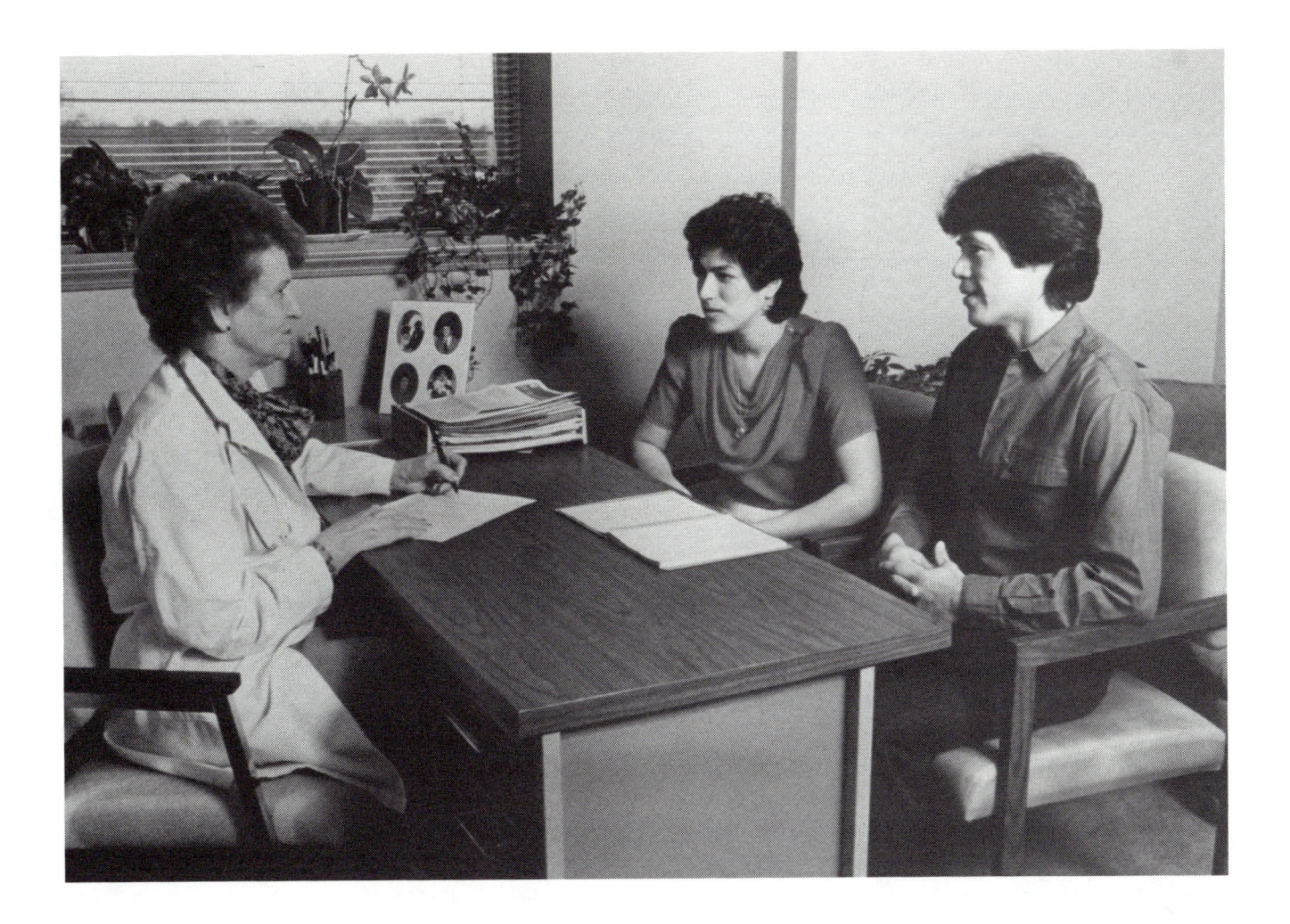

In diagnostic procedures, it may be used alone or in combination with amniocentesis (to increase safety and diagnostic accuracy); with fetoscopy (to allow accurate orientation of the fetoscope); and with radiographic techniques (to complement information for diagnosis). It is used in circumstances of elevated alpha-fetoprotein levels to rule out false positives and false negatives owing to inaccurate assessment of gestational age, fetal death, multiple pregnancy, and to define the abnormality present.

Fetoscopy and Fetal Blood Sampling

Using an instrument to view the fetus and obtaining fetal blood samples are considered necessary when information cannot be gathered by less risky or noninvasive methods and when the risk of the defect is considered "high." From this perspective, these procedures must be considered diagnostic rather than screening techniques. They allow diagnosis of genetic disorders of the skin that are not detectable by biochemical means; they provide a means of diagnosing blood disorders, such as sickle-cell anemia, thalassemia, and hemophilia A; and they allow the measurement of drugs and chemicals in tissues. In addition, these procedures can be used to verify many structural abnormalities and malformations.

A Sex-Linked Disease

Although the use of genetic screening procedures to determine sex of the unborn child is discouraged, such findings may encourage the termination of a pregnancy based on the reported incidence of a disease in one gender. All health care providers become involved directly and indirectly in such decisions. List criteria useful in these situations.

Alpha-Fetoprotein (AFP) and Acetylcholinesterase (AChE)

AFP can be detected in the amniotic fluid or in the maternal serum. An increase in AFP levels occurs not only in NTDs but also with other fetal anomalies. For this reason, it is considered a nonspecific test and thus can be utilized as a screening procedure. When both AFP and AChE levels are elevated, it increases accuracy in the diagnosis of NTDs. Moreover, when amniotic AFP, AChE, and ultrasound are used in combination, they create an accurate means of detecting NTDs.

Screening in Occupational Settings

Genetic screening in industry (via chromosome analysis) remains an option; however, both purpose and means have not been fully developed. The rationale for this type of screening includes:

* identifying those at greater risk than the average worker for suffering adverse effects from industrial exposure.

* detecting actual or potential damage of a genetic nature to presumed genetically "normal" workers.

Obviously, identification of high-risk populations must be completed, and the potential detrimental effects scrutinized. Such studies would require generational studies in most circumstances. Also of great concern is the development of reliable and inexpensive tests as well as the provision of the desired follow-up, follow-through, and/or treatment, all of which would be necessary if any program of screening is established.

Current Status of Mass Screening

Nationwide Practices

Practices vary according to state mandates and other variables. Sickle-cell screening, i.e., identification of carriers, which had been mandated in many states, was changed to a voluntary procedure. The federal government has funded carrier screening and genetic counseling. The geographic location of services associated with screening procedures has been a factor in determining whether specific states can utilize such procedures.

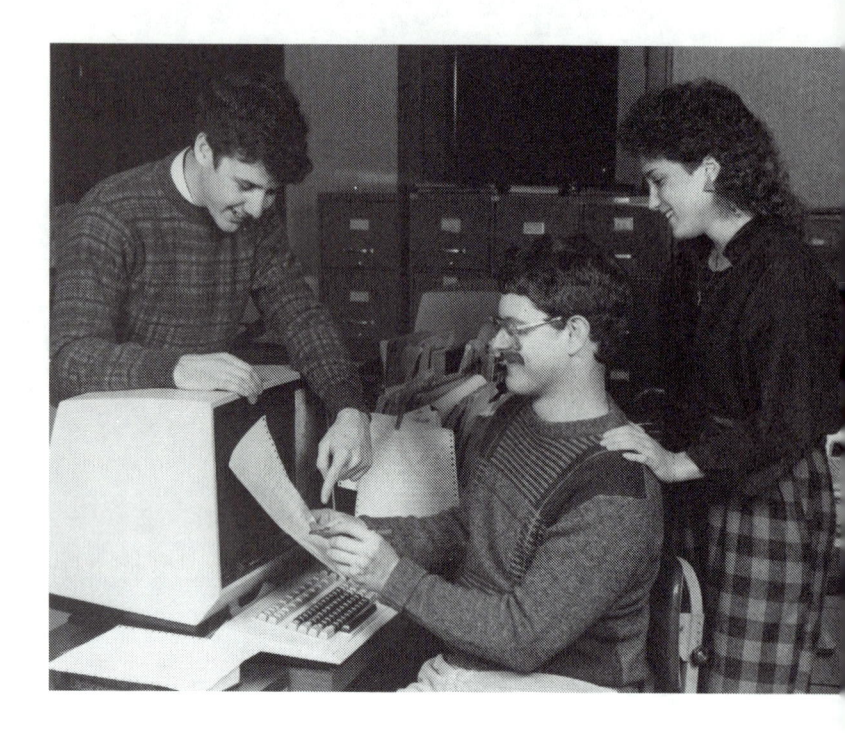

Information relating to screening of carriers and fetuses is not readily available, in part due to the voluntary status of such screening. However, in Texas, regional clinics provide such services. Also not available is information relating to screening in the workplace and the screening of donors. While such activities are ongoing, the findings are related to research and therefore limited in their applicability.

Texas Pattern

Because of the vastness of the state of Texas and the existence of identifiable high-risk groups there, it was decided to institute a comprehensive state program including eighteen regional clinics. Newborns were tested for congenital hypothyroidism, sickling hemoglobinopathies, phenylketonuria, and galactosemia. In 1985, 312,598 live births were reported (Althaus, 1986) and testing resulted in the diagnosis of:

* eight cases of phenylketonuria

* five cases of galactosemia

- ninety-four cases of congenital hypothyroidism
- ninety-two cases of sickle-cell disease

The significance of the regional clinics should be emphasized: clinical services must be available so that proper treatment can be given once a problem has been uncovered by genetic screening.

Ethical, Social, and Legal Issues

Clearly no discussion of the topic "Screening for Genetic Disorders" can be complete without a reminder that the moral, ethical, and legal aspects must be considered along with the scientific. Foremost in these considerations is *the right to refuse to participate;* even in compulsory situations, some states will exempt newborns from genetic screening if it violates the parents' religious beliefs. Genetic screening can produce some difficult to deal with findings such as "nonpaternity" and unexpected "incidental findings."

Much has been written about the ethical aspects of screening; however, only recently have ethics become a significant factor in decision making. Advances in technology will enable screening methods to increase and improve, but such knowledge must be used prudently and ethically. While global aspects of genetic screening cannot be denied, decisions must ultimately be made on an individual basis.

Currently, newborns constitute the largest group routinely screened. Funds for such screening are provided by state departments of health. These departments are faced with the stark realities of costs in fulfilling their obligations and must therefore base some decisions on financial rather than purely humanitarian terms. Data collected since the instigation of the screening of newborns for phenylketonuria give indisputable evidence of the value of this type of screening. The cost of screening and early treatment is small compared with the cost of long-term institutional care.

Screening to identify carriers is an essential component of genetic counseling. Genetic information on the individual and population groups provides the counselor with tools necessary to help the carrier and/or prospective parent make informed decisions. Carriers and noncarriers uniformly approve (96 percent) of genetic screening for themselves and for mutant genotypes; 92 percent of carriers and 95 percent of noncarriers approve of being screened in high school (Zessman, et al., 1984).

The Future of Screening for Genetic Defects

Three interrelated factors will influence the future of the practice: the need for screening, current outcomes, and new technologies.

The Need for Screening

As long as genetic disorders exist, the need for appropriate screening will be obvious. We must keep in mind that personal and religious values vary. Some persons identified as carriers may decide to have children. Some pregnancies involving fetuses determined to have serious defects will not be terminated. However, let us assume that more widespread prenatal screening will result in the identification of more disorders, and that more identification will result in more pregnancies being terminated, then the need for prenatal screening can be supported.

Public health reports confirm the relationship of congenital anomalies to infant deaths. For example, although there was a 41% reduction in infant deaths in 1980 as compared to 1960, "the absolute percentage of all infant deaths due to congenital anomalies had increased from 15.8% in 1960 to 24.1% in 1980" (Berry et al., 1987). In this study cardiovascular and central nervous system (CNS) anomalies accounted for 59% of infant deaths. At the present, cardiovascular anomalies are not as easily identified as CNS anomalies.

With improved methods, even more neural tube anomalies can be determined during prenatal screening. We cannot yet screen for the many conditions that seriously affect the quality of life and/or lead to death beyond the neonate period. However, risk factors of certain diseases in known carriers and maternal age groups suggest the need for extensive prenatal screening.

Current Outcomes

The detection of carriers among individuals of reproductive age may influence decisions to conceive children. For many, such decisions seem to be of less magnitude than decisions relating to the interruption of a pregnancy. Although screening is not diagnostic (in prenatal screening), it does provide the reasonable basis on which to pursue diagnosis and the possible termination of pregnancy. For many lay and science persons alike, this circumstance is clearly a dilemma.

The accompanying box presents excerpts from the policy statement of one organization relative to one particular kind of screening program, i.e., alpha-fetoprotein screening for neural tube defects.

While the screening process itself is relatively noncontroversial, certainly the results of the process may precipitate many dilemmas and difficult decisions. Health care providers must seek and obtain maximum patient input into decision making. Patients and providers should strive for mutual understanding, caring, and shared decision making.

While the decision to interrupt a pregnancy after diagnosing a possible congenital defect is primarily the woman's, a far larger group of individuals can be expected to influence that decision. In reaching a decision, the family should be well informed about "odds" and "risks" including the probability the present circumstance might occur in another pregnancy. A decision to interrupt a pregnancy may need to be made quickly due to the stage of development of the fetus but would never be made lightly as the couple must "live with that decision" for a long time. Genetic counseling of course has an important role in a couple's decision to conceive.

For many individuals of a variety of religious and cultural backgrounds, a decision to practice birth control or even achieve sterilization is far easier than interruption of pregnancy. Scientific information as a basis for decision making many times is taken lightly when a fundamental church doctrine and/or cultural attitude are involved.

New Technology

The knowledge base of and personal commitment to human genetics, including screening for genetic disorders, are expanding by quantum measures. Scriver (1987, p. 208), in a presidential address to the American Society of Human Genetics, cited a gain from "220 members in 1948 to just under 3000 in 1986." He also stated that approximately 2500 reports had been published describing more than 500 different human gene sequences in the ten years since the first cloned human gene was reported.

Contemporary literature and research publications alike discuss new developments relating to screening for genetic disorders such as diabetes mellitus and cystic fibrosis.

Rotter and Rimoin (1987) concluded that diabetes mellitus is inherited in some sense (it runs in families)

Maternal Serum Alpha-Fetoprotein Screening

POLICY STATEMENT EXCERPTS
AMERICAN SOCIETY OF HUMAN GENETICS

Maternal serum alpha-fetoprotein (MSAFP) values are used primarily but not solely to predict occurrence of open neural tube defects in the fetus; their use for prediction of Down's syndrome is a new initiative under investigation. Because there is no effective treatment to relax the burden of neural tube defects in the large majority of patients, at the present time prevention of disease involves termination of pregnancy. In other words, use of the test is value laden and controversial for some sectors of society. MSAFP screening is a screening test and is not diagnostic. MSAFP screening should be voluntary.

Before the specimen for MSAP testing is obtained, the patient should have been fully informed about the procedure and its implications and should indicate her willingness to be tested. For religious and ethic reasons, some couples may not want to be confronted with the dilemmas posed by an abnormal test result. Prenatal MSAFP screening should be voluntary. The provider should indicate its availability, educate the patient about its potential, and allow the patient to make decisions concerning participation in screening and in the sequential steps in the management of pregnancies. The patient's decision on whether or not to have MSAFP screening should be documented by such means as her written signature.

American Journal of Human Genetics

---

although its inheritance rarely follows any simple Mendelian pattern. However, the same authors predict that, in another ten years, our ability to identify individuals at risk and circumvent the consequences should improve markedly.

In the case of suspected cystic fibrosis in the fetus, studies by Mulivor et al. (1987) indicate the possibility of effective screening. An arbitrary cutoff point could be chosen for three enzymes (amniotic-fluid intestinal alkaline phosphatase, gamma-glutamyltranspeptidase,

> **Fetus with Fetal Condition**
>
> Genetic screening of newborns for PKU has become common practice and is readily accepted by parents. One reason, of course, is the fact that treatment is available. However, there are many other inherited conditions for which treatment is not readily available. Discuss the ethical issues related to informing patients that genetic screening of their newborn has detected a condition that has no known cure and is usually fatal..

and leucine-aminopeptidase) that would enable one to correctly predict the outcome for many at-risk pregnancies.

Although currently used for diagnostic purposes, the **scrutiny of chorionic villi** is among the new technologies that have potential for screening as well. At least one researcher (Gustavii, 1984) supports chorionic villi sampling under direct vision because it can be done at an earlier stage than amniocentesis. Certainly, amniocentesis is far more commonly used. Most amniotic fluids, whatever the primary reason for amniocentesis, are tested to determine the presence of fetal anencephaly or open spina bifida.

Dacus et al. (1985), reporting on twelve years of genetic amniocentesis reaffirmed its potential as a screening device. The authors conclude that in 2000 patients, one percent had aneuploid fetuses (one having an abnormal number of chromosomes) and another one percent had elevated amniotic fluid concentrations of alpha-fetoprotein.

A relevant *Newsweek* column appeared with the title "Cause for Concern – and Optimism" and the subtitle "Of every 100 babies, three have major defects." The author, Jerry Adler (1987), summarizes the current situation, charging that the rate of birth defects has changed little since the time when such statistics started to be gathered (1960):

While there is no doubt that drugs, radiation, and environmental pollutants can cause birth defects in individual cases, statistically they don't seem to have contributed to much of an increase. But then neither have the great advances in genetics and embryology in the last 20 years brought about a noticeable decrease. If the majority of birth defects are the result of natural genetic variation – the price we pay, one might speculate, for the gifts of evolution – then there are no easy or obvious ways for medicine to eradicate them.

Adler claims that research has been spotty and that no cures have been found for conditions such as Down's syndrome. Presenting information relating to environmentally caused birth defects, he writes:

But most of the proven cases of environmentally caused birth defects (exclusive of alcohol and drug abuse) appear to fall into three categories; infectious disease (in the United States, chiefly cytomegalovirus, a generally mild flulike infection); drugs that are essential to a woman's health and taken in awareness of their risk (certain anticonvulsants and anticoagulants), and drugs taken by women who do not know they are pregnant.

Adler concludes on a pessimistic note:

This is progress, of course, but progress of a discouragingly slow and piecemeal kind. It tells one small group of mothers why their children were born defective, compounding their grief with the certain knowledge that they brought this tragedy on their children themselves. For the rest, medicine offers only the cold consolation of ignorance.

Most researchers seem to have a more optimistic point of view. Kan et al. (1987) writes:

The availability of recombinant DNA probes has vastly increased the scope of prenatal diagnosis of genetic disorders. Random DNA probes may soon be used to diagnose diseases in which the defective structural gene has not been identified. In addition, the isolation of Y-chromosome-specific probes has provided a rapid method of fetal sex determination, and early diagnosis of genetic disorders in the first trimester is being explored using chorionic villi biopsy.

Undoubtedly a twentieth-century development, "mass screening for genetic disorders" will not have its full impact until the twenty-first century.

Summary

Screening for genetic disorders constitutes a modern miracle made possible by interdisciplinary research. Scientists have developed and continue to develop screening procedures, which are becoming more widely used in both mandatory and voluntary circumstances. Today newborns constitute the largest, most easily identified group that are routinely screened. Prenatal screening is increasing, whereas detection of carriers calls for screening large numbers of men and women of reproductive age. Potential donors in artificial insemination programs are screened to verify their genetic status. Occupational (workplace) screening is a response to the scientific community's increasing awareness of toxic agents and their presumed detrimental effect on genes.

Screening programs remain relatively expensive. However, there are both identified and presumed evidences that screening with concurrent treatment has saved society many dollars in institutional care. The availability of treatment and genetic counseling are both significant factors in providing screening. Although the history of genetic screening is short (only twenty-five years), the achievements are remarkable and the future promises more procedures will become available.

Cited References

Adler, J. Cause for concern – and optimism. (1987, March 16). *Newsweek,* 63-66.

Althaus, B. (1986, October 24). Personal communication.

Berry, R. J., et al. (1987). Birth weight-specific infant mortality due to congenital anomalies, 1960-1980. *Public Health Reports,* 102, (2): 171-77.

Brock, D. J. H. Amniotic fluid tests for fetal neural tube defects. (1983). *British Medical Bulletin,* 39 (4): 373-77.

Cohen, F. L. (1984). *Clinical genetics in nursing practice.* Philadelphia: Lippincott.

Dacus, J. V., et al. (1985). Genetic amniocentesis; a twelve years' experience. *American Journal of Medical Genetics,* 20 (3): 443-52.

Fletcher, J. C. (1984). Ethical and social aspects of risk predictions, *Clinical Genetics,* 25 (4): 25-31.

Gustavii, B. (1984). Chorionic villi sampling under direct vision. *Clinical Genetics,* 26 (4): 297-300.

Kan, Y. W., et al. (1987). Genetics diagnosis by DNA analysis. Advances in Gene Technology: Human Genetic Disorders, *Cambridge: Cambridge University Press,* pp. 79-81.

Meany, J. L. (1985, April). *Screening for genetic disorders,* Lecture presented at Indiana University Medical School, Indianapolis.

Mulivor, R. A., et al. (1987). Analysis of fetal intestinal enzymes in amniotic fluid for the prenatal diagnosis of cystic fibrosis, *American Journal of Human Genetics,* 40: 13-46.

Murray, R. F. (1986). Tests of so-called genetic susceptibility; conference on medical screening and biological monitoring for the effects of exposure in the workplace. *Journal of Occupational Medicine,* 28 (10): 1103-7.

Newill, C., et al. (1986). Epidemiological approach to the evaluation of genetic screening in the workplace; conference on medical screening and biological monitoring for the effects of exposure in the workplace. *Journal of Occupational Medicine,* 28 (10): 1108-11.

Rotter, J. I., and Rimoin, D. I. (1987, May 15). The genetics of diabetes, *Hospital Practice,* 81-88.

Rowley, P. T., et al. (1984). Genetic screening, marvel or menace? *Science,* 225:138-44.

Scriver, C.R. (1987). Presidential address; physiological genetics – who needs it? *American Journal of Human Genetics,* 40: 199-211.

Zessman, S., et al. (1984). A private view of heterozygosity; eight year follow-up study on carriers of Tay-Sachs gene detected by high school screening in Montreal. *American Journal of Medical Genetics,* 1 (4): pp 769-775.

Sickle-Cell Anemia

Mary and Joe have a whirlwind courtship. Mary marries Joe without telling him that she has sickle-cell disease. Soon after their first child is born, Joe discovers that he has the same disease. The couple go for counseling to find out what problems might arise if they should have additional children. In spite of the fact that they both have active sickle-cell disease, Mary and Joe decide to have another child.

- Should sickle-cell screening be mandatory upon applying for a marriage license?

- Should Mary and Joe have been allowed to marry?

- Having discovered that Joe has the disease also, should they be allowed to have more children?

- Does society have a responsibility to help Mary and Joe with medical bills that could result from this disease?

- Should society demand sterilization of couples such as Mary and Joe?

- If you know you have a negative genetic trait, should you be sterilized or refrain from having children?

- Should amniocentesis, genetic counseling, and even abortion be mandatory upon discovering a pregnant woman has a negative genetic trait?

- When do you think someone should tell a prospective mate that he/or she has a negative genetic trait?

- Should there be mass screening for genetic disorders? If yes, who should conduct such screenings and when should they be administered?

- Who should pay for a mass screening program if one is desired?

- Should any health care be offered to a person with a genetic defect? If so, how much should be given?

- Do parents have a "right" to try to have a child on the off-chance that there will be no genetic problems?

- Should other people have to pay for the care of an infant born to parents who knew they had genetic problems but conceived a child anyway?

- How would you feel if you were told that you had a problem such as sickle-cell anemia or Tay-Sachs disease?

8

Issues and Problems of Organ Transplantation

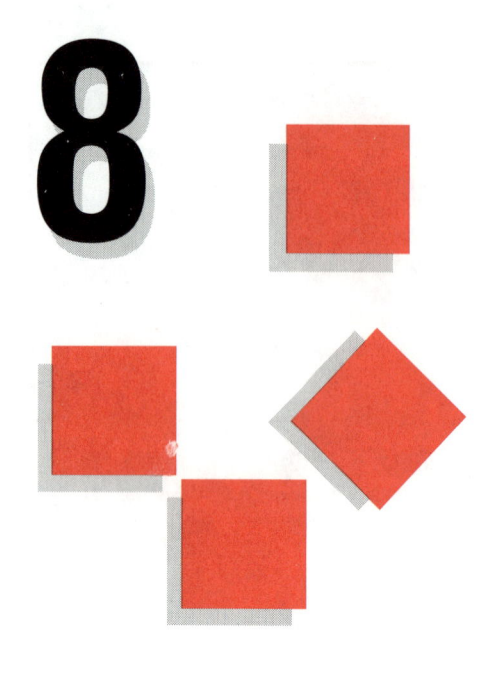

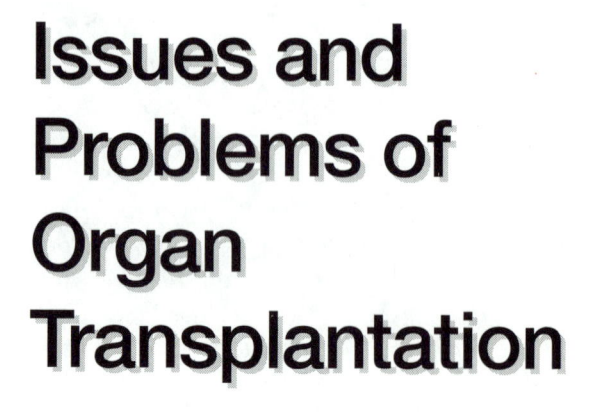

Janice R. Sandiford*

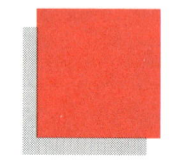

Objectives

After reading this chapter, you should be able to:

- Define the terms listed at the beginning of this chapter.
- Discuss how the practice of organ transplantation evolved in the United States.
- Identify the factors that contribute to the high cost of organ transplantation.
- Discuss the legal restrictions imposed on organ transplantation.
- Identify religious and ethnic views on organ transplantation.
- Describe the referral process for obtaining organs.
- Identify agencies involved in coordinating and obtaining organs for transplantation.

Terms and Definitions

Cadaver organ. Body part taken from a corpse.
Genetically identical. Having the same hereditary character structure.
Harvesting. Gathering organs for transplanting to others.
Immunosuppressive drugs. Medications used to reduce the opportunity for rejection to occur.
Procurement. Obtaining organs.

Introduction

The medical community began transplanting organs in the mid 1960s. In the past 10 years, many organ transplant procedures have changed from experimental procedures to routine therapeutic interventions. Hardly a day goes by that the media does not carry a story about organ transplants. Some are successful; some are not. Some are performed on infants, some on individuals beyond middle age. Some types of transplants are still experimental and success rates unpredictable. Even with major advances in technology, people continue to die while waiting for a matched donor. In spite of advances in immunosuppressive drug therapy, situations occur that effect the long-term prognosis of individuals with transplanted organs. Despite the ever-increasing use of organ transplantation, issues and problems exist relative to the practice, both legal and ethical.

Health care professionals are, and will continue to be, members of transplant teams and will care for individuals, both recipients and donors. Legal questions have been raised about the transplant programs and most are somewhat easy to deal with. Ethical questions, however, are not quite as easy. Many ethical questions are still unanswered. It is imperative that health care professionals discuss their feelings with other practitioners. This chapter is written to help you discuss some of these issues and problems. Through your discussion, it is hoped that you will begin to formulate your opinions on this topic. As a health care provider, you will be asked to assist others in making decisions. You should know where your beliefs lie, and you should know the facts.

---

*Janice R. Sandiford
Associate Professor, Health Occupations Education, College of Education, Florida International University, North Miami Campus, N. Miami, FL 33181.

Quality of Life

A major issue of concern is quality of life. This is a matter that must be carefully considered by the prospective recipient, or by the parents when the patient is a minor. Will life with the new organ be better than life without it? Will pain be eased? Will complications be minimal? To live a life tethered to the medical system may not be the life of choice. There is also the risk of failure that must be reckoned with: If the transplant fails, what will life be like?

When transplants were a new procedure, success rates were not very high. As the success rates improved, the quality of life issues become more important.

In the early years, the survival rate after kidney transplantation was relatively low; only about 28 percent of those who received transplants of kidneys from cadavers survived two years (Katz and Capron, 1975). Today, the rate is approaching 95 percent. The highest success rate occurs when the kidney is provided by a live donor. There is a 72 percent chance for survival one year after transplantation when sibling donors are used, and a 66 percent chance when parents are the donors (Renal Transplant Registry).

In heart transplantation, one-year survival rates are being reported at 81 percent, and five-year survival rates are well over 50 percent (Friedrich, 1984; Raithel, 1987, and Wood et al., 1987). Schroeder and Hunt (1987) found some centers reporting 100% survival rates after one year. Success rates for liver transplants are at 65-70 percent (Friedrich, 1984), with liver recipients up to 16 years of age having an 80% chance of surviving the first year (Wood et al., 1987). The improved rates reflect the development and use of immunosuppressive drugs, such as cyclosporine, which keep the body from rejecting the new foreign organ.

Quality of life and successful rehabilitation have improved steadily for those receiving heart transplants from cadavers. Stanford (1986) reports that 85 percent of patients who have survived for one year have been able to make free choices about what to do with their lives, with some returning to full-time employment.

The recipient of a transplant must be on the alert that the new organ is not rejected by the body. To ward off this danger, **immunosuppressive drugs** are given to the patient for the remainder of his or her life. Rejection is greatest during the first three months and usually decreases with time. Often several drugs are necessary with the goal to maintain effective immunosuppression with the lowest possible doses without toxicity.

The greatest complication of immunosuppression therapy is increased susceptibility to infection which may require treatment with toxic agents. Long-term immunosuppressive therapy can also lead to the development of lymphatic malignancies, skeletal demineralization, glucose intolerance, nephrotoxicity and difficult to manage hypertension. But despite such concerns and regimens, the quality of life will generally be enhanced by the successful transplant.

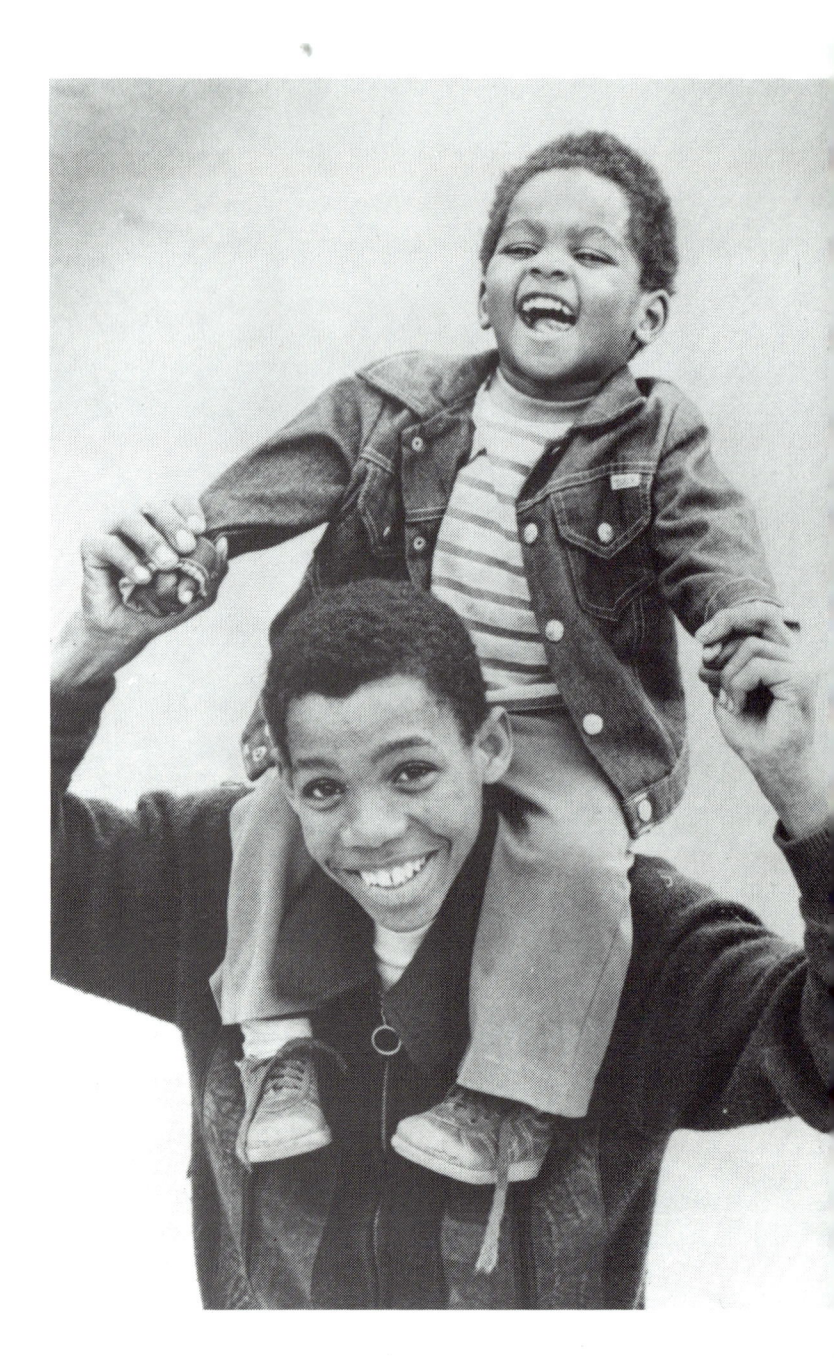

Cost of Transplantation

Another major issue is cost of the transplant and liability for payment. The risks of organ transplants are great enough that the cost is exorbitant.

Surgery to transplant a kidney may cost as much as $30,000, whereas surgery to transplant a heart might be $200,000. A patient can run up expenses of $250,000 before getting a liver transplant, then pay $135,000 for the transplant, followed by a year of rehabilitation costing $135,000. Bone marrow transplants run to $60,000. Immunosuppressive therapy costs $500 per month.

Liability insurance for medical personnel and the medical facility must be considered in the total cost of a transplant. They need to be protected from malpractice suits, and the cost of such protection gets passed back to the health care consumer.

Third party payers, typically insurance companies and the government, have been forced to establish limits of payment: $107,000 for heart, $129,000 for heart-lung, and $240,000 for liver. Insurance firms generally decline payment for operations involving newer technology (heart, heart-lung, and liver) on the grounds that they are still experimental. Blue Cross of California began a new era by paying for heart transplants in early 1984 (Friedrich, 1984). By 1986, heart transplantation was no longer considered experimental and was covered by most major health insurance programs providing the possibility of transplantation for those with insurance. Medicare began coverage for individuals under fifty-five years of age who were ineligible for other insurance coverage, thus making it possible for even the poor to have a chance. Kidney transplants are more acceptable; insurance companies are willing to pay $40,000 for a transplant rather than provide about $18,000 per year to maintain a patient on dialysis.

What, then, becomes of the remaining costs? In 1972, the federal government decided to pay 80 percent of the cost of kidney transplants and dialysis for patients whose kidneys fail. The first year's bill came to $241 million for 10,300 patients, with expectations of soaring increases to 82,000 patients in the 1980s (Friedrich,

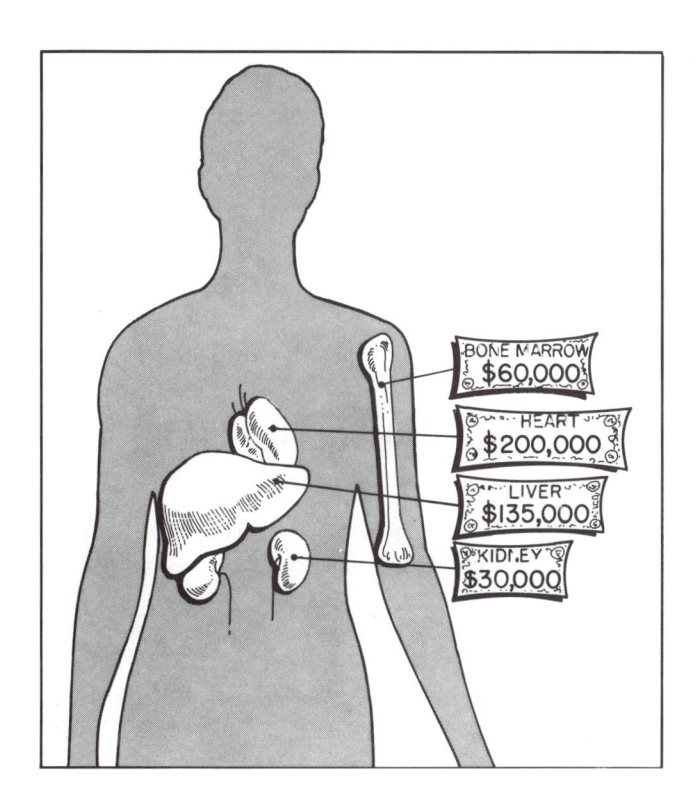

Organ Transplantation

The Mercedes family has set of identical twins, John and James. At eight years of age both children came down with chickenpox. As a result, James developed encephalitis which left him brain damaged. John was luckier than James. He was left with a residual kidney problem. John attended regular school while James went to special classes. At home, James frequently had temper tantrums. He threw things and even attempted to hurt himself. John, on the other hand, was well liked, an excellent student, and an outstanding athlete.

In his physical for college, it is discovered that John's kidneys are starting to fail, and a kidney transplant will be needed to save his life. Further testing reveals that the only compatible donor is his brother James.

What action should be taken and why?

1984). In the Medicare program it is estimated that by 1991, payments for about 140 heart transplants will be close to $25 million. Even with Medicare reimbursement, hospitals stand to lose $20,000 per transplant as reimbursement falls short of actual costs. Since we don't know whether the government can continue to cover such expenses over the long run, the burden for payment may be placed on the recipient (or the family). In this case, perhaps only the rich can be recipients. The bill for William Schroeder's artificial heart operation and treatment would have covered 113 patients for an average week in the hospital! The bill for a liver transplant could operate an inner-city clinic, providing 30,000 office visits for one year (Friedrich, 1984).

Does Organ Transplantation Discriminate Against the Old and the Poor

Organ transplants tend to be limited to a specific age group. Kidneys are usually not transplanted to individuals over the age of fifty-five, and the unofficial cut-off age for heart transplants is fifty years. However, it is difficult to determine when, if, or how often medical service has been denied. But is it moral to deny someone a transplant simply on the basis of age, when the procedure can save a life?

It is anticipated that fewer than 100 patients a year will qualify for Medicare reimbursement for heart transplants (Lutz, 1988). It's an old saying that "money talks." Those that have it have more access to transplants than those who do not. Since there just are not enough organs to go around and the cost of transplantation is so great, will there come a time when only the rich will receive transplants?

Research: Issues of Time, Money, and Regulation

A considerable amount of time is required in research before experimentation can begin on humans. Take, as an example, the development of kidney transplantation. The first such transplantation in laboratory animals was reported in 1902, the first human trial in 1947 (for a short-term problem using a cadaver organ). But it was not until 1954 that a genetically identical donor kidney was implanted into a sibling (Katz and Capron, 1975). In many cases of organ transplant, we are still researching the techniques. Physicians, especially surgeons, must be trained in transplant procedures as well as in techniques of follow-up care. Where does the training take place? Who pays while physicians learn? Does this training require human subjects?

Before 1970, there was little federal regulation of health care. Today this is not so. In 1979, the administrative authority for Medicare and Medicaid (Health Care Financing Administration) authorized payment for experimental heart transplantation done on Medicare patients at Stanford University Medical Center. But in June 1980 this authority put a stop to such payments until a review of new health care technologies took place. Selection criteria were established, and six study centers were reimbursed for fifteen heart transplants (Creighton, 1985, Friedrich, 1984).

The process was too slow, however, causing medical centers to seek other funding sources such as teaching funds and grants.

By 1987, 117 hospitals were performing heart transplants, with fifteen hospitals having qualified for Medicare reimbursement. Seeking certification as a Medicare heart transplant center is not easy. Hospitals are required to perform 36 transplants within three years (Lutz, 1988).

All this experimentation costs money and valuable time. In the meantime, many of those who may have benefited from transplantation have died from their illness.

◆ First Transplant

In the first human trial of renal transplantation, the patient had not urinated for ten days, was in a deep coma, and was not expected to live (Katz and Capron, 1975). Fortunately, the physicians ignored the hospital's objections and did the transplantation, which had positive results. This is not always the case.

What Criteria Should Be Used in Deciding on a Transplant?

The individual should make an informed decision on whether to agree to an organ transplantation. But when in a constant state of poor health or pain, a person may be easily influenced by others who are in a position of authority and who speak with confidence. The person may blindly accept a physician's advice, and even treatment plans that may be selfish or questionable, without seeking a second opinion. Many are at the end of their rope and vulnerable.

As far as the medical community is concerned, it generally reserves transplants for those patients with the bleakest prognosis. Patients who require cardiac transplantation have reached a point where no medical regimen or conventional surgical procedure will improve or alter the progress of their disease. They must undergo clinical and laboratory studies to rule out serious pulmonary hypertension, psychological deficiencies, active infection, or other systemic disease that would complicate recovery. Then a committee must unanimously agree that no lesser surgical procedure would be beneficial and that the patient would not survive six months unless a transplant was done.

Likewise, kidney transplant patients have undergone years of dialysis, with treatments three to four times per week. Their quality of life is limited by frequent trips to the dialysis unit.

The Issue of Supply and Demand

Despite the proliferation of transplants, the demand is still greater than the supply. In 1984, 7,000 kidneys, 350 hearts, 300 livers, 90 pancreases, and 25 heart-lungs were transplanted (Whitman, 1985). In 1986, 8,973 kidneys, 1,368 hearts, 924 livers, 140 pancreases, and 45 heart-lungs were transplanted (Lutz, 1988). During early 1986, the North American Transplant Coordinators Organization estimated that thousands are waiting for transplants: 8,000 for kidneys, 500 for livers, 400 for hearts, 100 for heart-lungs, 3,000-5,000 for corneas, 200 for pancreases, and 100,000 for tissue, bone, and skin.

By 1987, the numbers awaiting transplants had risen to 9,000 for kidneys, 300 for hearts, 75 for heart-lungs,

Major Events in Organ Transplant History

1954   First living-related donor kidney transplant performed at Brigham Hospital, Boston, Massachusetts.

1962   First post-mortem kidney transplant performed at Brigham.

1967   Christiaan Barnard, M.D., performs first heart transplant in Capetown, South Africa.

Thomas Starzl, M.D., performs first liver transplant at University of Colorado.

1981   First heart-lung transplant at Stanford University.

1982   Barney Clark receives first permanent artificial heart at University of Utah.

1983   The anti-rejection drug, cyclosporine, is approved by the FDA.

1984   At request of U.S. Surgeon General, Dr. Starzl publishes instructions on procuring organs other than kidneys. Procedure later became known as Pittsburgh technique.

National Organ Transplant Act signed into law establishing a national system to match donors and recipients.

1986   United Network for Organ Sharing (UNOS), Richmond, Virginia, awarded federal contract to ensure equitable access and allocation of organs. UNOS begins setting membership criteria and standards for transplant centers.

1987   A new Federal law requires hospitals to approach relatives of brain-dead patients about organ donation.

Medicare begins paying for heart transplants at hospitals that meet survival and experience criteria set by the Health Care Financing Administration (HCFA).

HCFA certifies organ procurement agencies.

300 for livers, 50 for pancreases, and 5,000 for corneas (Lutz, 1988).

Another estimate is that of 15,000 people per year who need heart transplants, only 200 get them. It has been estimated that as many as 30,000 Americans could benefit from heart transplants, but only 7,000 to 8,000 hearts are likely to be available in any year – and 60 percent of those are lost because they object to transplantation or are ignorant about the procedure (Naunton, 1986). In one study of twenty-six potential donors, only eight donations actually took place.

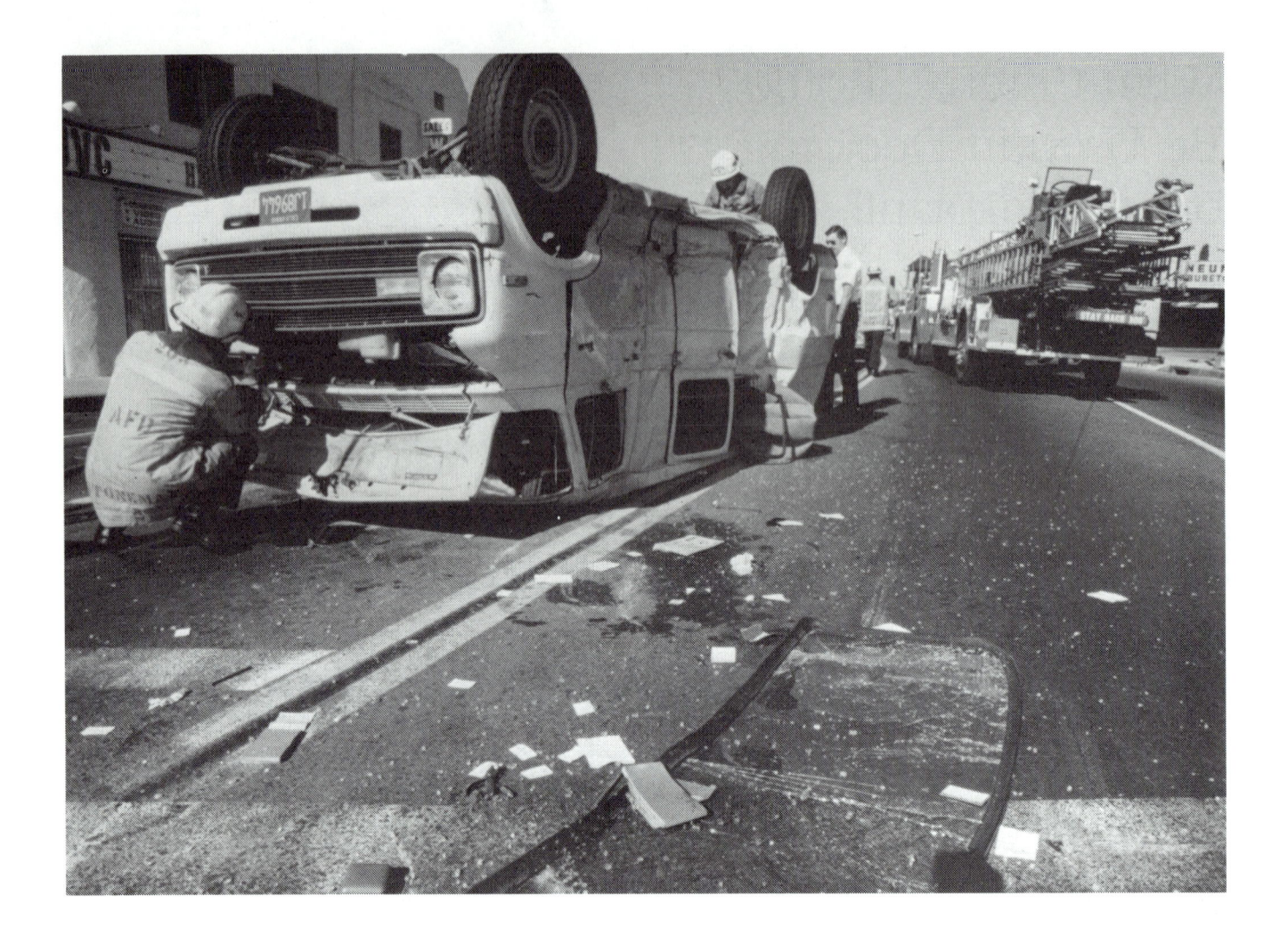

Not all organs are suitable for transplantation. The age range of most suitable liver and kidney donors is newborn to fifty years of age (Williams, 1985), whereas hearts of donors are generally between fifteen and forty years of age. Donors of small size can create technical problems in organ removal, and donors weighing more than 200 pounds are rarely suitable for reasonable matches (Williams).

Other factors may influence the availability of organs. Even if a person has signed a donor card, organs are generally not removed without written permission from the next of kin – out of respect for the donor family's wishes (Creighton, 1985, Malecki, 1986). Blacks are less likely than whites to want their own kidney donated – 10 percent vs. 27 percent (Koop, 1983).

On the other hand, those who have completed more years of formal education and those in the higher

Transplants Performed in the U.S.

Organ or Tissue	1981	1982	1983	1984	1985	1986	Numbers awaiting transplants 1987
Kidney	4,885	5,358	6,162	6,968	7,695	8,973	9,000
Heart	62	103	172	346	731	1,368	300
Heart/Lung	5	7	20	22	30	45	75
Liver	26	62	164	308	605	924	300
Pancreas	_	35	61	87	133	140	50
Cornea	_	18,500	21,250	24,000	26,326	31,000	5,000
Bone	475	800	990	1,000	1,200	1,160	Marrow _

Figures are approximate numbers for certain organs and tissue transplants and for those medically approved and actually awaiting

income brackets are more likely to want their own organs donated. And in a study of ten families who were offered the chance to donate organs, eight of them did so (Williams, 1985): thus, being informed about the procedure appears to have a positive influence.

The demand for organs is clear; the supply, however, is dependent on the willingness of individuals to donate organs to others. Often death is a prerequisite for donation; then the decision becomes one that the next of kin must deal with. How many of you have signed an organ donation card or identified yourself as an organ donor on your driver's license? (Automobile accidents are the most common source of donated organs.) Do you plan to let this decision be made by those you leave behind?

Deciding to "Pull the Plug"

Pulling the plug! Do you agree to pull life-support systems so that another unrelated and unknown individual can benefit? As health care professionals, we are often faced with the task of encouraging families to make this decision. When has death occurred – when the brain ceases to function or when the heart stops circulating blood? Could you make the decision to pull life supports from your wife/husband, son/daughter, mother/father? How do you learn to live with your decision and accept it?

The fact that no major religious group (Catholic, Jewish, Protestant) prohibits organ donation (Creighton, 1985) should prove reassuring for those considering donation of organs of a loved one.

Also to be noted is that organ donation does not mean body mutilation. The surgery is done using a standard sterile environment in an operating room (Malecki, 1986).

The longer a donor stays on life support, the less likely the organs will be in condition for transplant (Weber, 1985). So even though the decision in favor of organ donation is a difficult one, time is of the essence.

Complications Related to Transplantation

Organ transplantation is high risk! Although success rates have increased remarkably since the first transplants, the risk of complications still exists. The major concern is life or death, but other problems may occur such as minimum organ function, rejection, infection, pain. Can the abilities of the medical team counteract all possible complications? Will they identify them in time to prevent unacceptable consequences?

Some hard facts:

- The average increase in the lives of heart transplant patients is only three years (Friedrich, 1984).
- There is evidence that immunosuppressive drugs can increase the likelihood of cancer.
- Half of an average person's lifetime medical expenses will occur during the last six months of life (Friedrich, 1984).
- Organ recipients must "change their lifestyle."

Unethical Practices

Although it may seem a little bizarre, unethical practices are indeed real possibilities. Professionals could counsel families to prematurely disconnect life support in search of donor organs. Body snatching could exist, particularly of individuals who list no next of kin. Death could be premature as induced by medication. And although it's illegal to buy and sell body organs (National Organ Procurement Act, 1984), money could encourage people to donate them.

- The longest kidney transplant survivor is a twin who received a transplant over twenty years ago (Katz and Capron, 1975).
- In heart transplantation, an individual has an 80 percent chance of living for one year, and a 75 percent chance of living for five years.

Summary

This topic is certainly one that should establish dialogue among health care professionals and students. We need to begin to take action. There is a need to develop standards for medical and nursing care of donors and recipients, to encourage publications focusing on transplantation, and for collaborative programming. As a new health professional, you will be in a position to set precedent or even to become involved in establishing standards.

In this chapter, you have had the opportunity to consider some of the issues of organ transplantation. You have also had an opportunity to examine your beliefs about organ transplantation. Right or wrong – who knows! As we develop more sophistication in the technology of organ transplantation, we may be able to answer this question.

Cited References

Carosella, J. (1984). Picking up the pieces: the unsuccessful kidney transplant. *Health Social Work,* 9 (2): 142-43.

Creighton, H. (1985). Organ transplantation (part 1). *Nursing Management,* 16 (9): 16, 18.

Creighton, H. (1985). Organ transplantation (part 2). *Nursing Management,* 16 (10): 20, 22.

Friedrich, O. (1984). One miracle, many doubts. *Time,* 124 (24): 70-73, 77.

Garibaldi, R. A. (1983). Infections in organ transplant recipients. *Infection Control,* 4 (6): 460-64.

Geller, T. (1986). Organ procurement: nurses have a vital role to play. *RNabe News,* 18 (1): 8-11.

Jader, G. (1985). Second chance . . . agree to a heart transplant or die. (case study). *American Journal of Nursing,* 85 (5): 568K-L, 568N.

Katz, J., and Capron, A. M. (1975). Issues in kidney transplantations. Adapted from *Catastrophic diseases: who decides what? a psychosocial and legal analysis of the problems posed by hemodialysis and organ transplantation.* By Jay Katz and Alexander Morgan Capron, New York: Russell Sage Foundation, 1975, pp. 39-51.

Koop, C. E. (1983). Increasing the supply of solid organs for transplantation. *Public Health Report,* 98 (6): 566-72.

Lutz, S. (1988). Organ transplant programs multiply. *Modern Healthcare,* March 4, 1988, pp. 23-31.

Malecki, M. S. (1986). A personal perspective: working with families who donate organs and tissues. *AORN Journal,* 44 (1): 44-47.

Naunton, Ena. (1986, August 12). Transplant business is booming. *The Miami Herald,* pp. 1C, 3C.

Raithel, K. S. (1987) 20 Years after first human heart transplant, 1987 may see 4000 procedures performed worldwide. *Journal of the American Medical Association,* 258 (21): 3084-3085.

Rosen, L. (1985). Medical-legal issues associated with organ donation and transplantation: living donors (part 2). *Today's OR Nurse,* 7 (8): 32-33.

Schroeder, J.S., and Hunt, S., Cardiac transplantation: Update 1987. *Journal of the American Medical Association.* 258 (21) 3142-3145.

Skelly, L. (1985). Practical issues in obtaining organs for transplantation. *Law Medical Health Care,* 13 (1): 35-37.

Solomon, S. B. (1985). Organ transplant law raises thorny questions. *Nursing & Health Care,* 6 (1): 19-20.

Stanford, T.M., (1986). The potential organ donor. *Emergency,* 18 (3): 36-39.

Weber, P. (1985). The human connection: the role of the nurse in organ donation. *Journal of Neurosurgical Nursing,* 17 (2): 119-22.

Whitman, D. (1985). Transplanting life . . . organ transplants. *US News and World Report,* 99 (23): 66-67.

Williams, L. (1985). Organ procurement: what nurses need to know. CCQ, 8 (1): 27-30.

Wood, C., Lowther, W., Surette, R., and Smith, D. (1987). The transplant revolution. *Maclean's,* 100: 34-40.

Liver Transplant

A young girl is brought to a metropolitan medical center suffering from child abuse. Her liver is so severely damaged that a transplant is essential to save her life. Livers are difficult to obtain for transplant, and no liver is available. The child's name is put on a waiting list, with the hope that a liver becomes available before she dies.

During this time a second child, Arthur, is admitted with a liver problem. This child also will require a transplant within a few months to a year. Arthur has been admitted so that some additional tests can be done. His parents are quite wealthy and are doing everything they can to care for him.

Around 7:00 p.m. there is a severe accident and a young child is brought to the emergency room with multiple head injuries. Arthur's parents hear about the accident and that a child about Arthur's age is dying. They contact the parents and offer them a large cash settlement for their child's liver.

- How should the decision be made as to which child should get the liver?

- Should medical need dictate who gets the liver?

- Would the little girl who has been physically abused have excessive psychological damage that would need attention? Would this influence the decision?

- When people have money, and try to use it to help their child, should that be held against them?

- If a child of yours or another member of your family were in a similar situation, would you use every means to keep your child alive?

- Suppose the parents of the dead child have limited finances and could use the money. Do they have any moral or ethical obligations?

- If one of the candidates for the liver were mentally incompetent, would that influence the decision about who should get the liver?

- Suppose, instead of mental incompetence, one of the children has physical disabilities. Would that make a difference?

- If the deceased child were mentally deficient, in what way might this affect the decision of the parents?

- Is this a decision that should be decided by the court?

- Should people with money be prohibited from advertising for needed organs?

- Should someone be able to sell an organ for transplant?

- Would the medical staff take "better" care of a child who has well-to-do parents than one from a poverty-level family?

- If the child whom the staff thought didn't deserve the liver actually was transplanted, would the quality of care be influenced?

- If the dead child had been a nonwhite, would there have been as much willingness to transplant the liver?

- If one of the children who needed the liver were white and the other nonwhite, would this influence which child was transplanted?

- Suppose the transplanted liver was rejected by the child's body. Should the next available liver go to that child or the next person in line?

- Would a sizable sum offered for an organ tend to increase the availability of donors?

- Should organs be transplanted from one body to another?

9

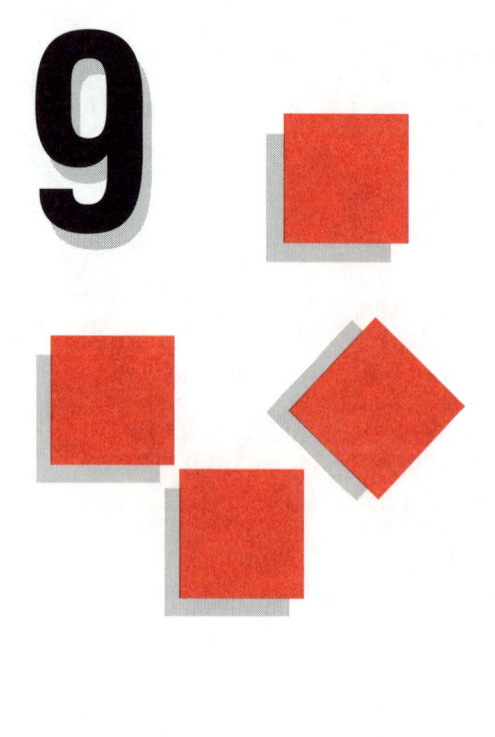

Scientific Knowledge Versus Human Experimentation

Norma Jean Schira*

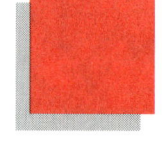

Objectives

After reading this chapter, you should be able to:
- Define the terms listed at the beginning of this chapter.
- Explain informed consent as it relates to research involving human subjects.
- Discuss the common moral and ethical questions related to research, experimentation, and technology.
- Differentiate between practice and research.
- Explain the ways that guidelines for biomedical research protect subjects involved with the research.
- Discuss the importance and/or relationship of protection of human subjects and biomedical ethics.

Terms and Definitions

Autonomy/Autonomous. Independent/self-governing. Makes decisions and determines goals and choices.
Beneficence. Risk versus gains or benefits.
Incapacitated. Unable to be independent, make decisions, or determine goals or choices.
Justice. Equal chance of selection, cannot provide undue rewards or benefits for participation.
Nuremburg Code. Guidelines and standards for determining scientific and ethical conduct of physicians and scientists who were involved with abuses of and criminal acts performed on human subjects in the concentration camps during World War II.
Placebo. An inactive substance used in research to test effectiveness of a particular drug or treatment.

Introduction

Drug experimentation is a term used to cover the broad area of experiments or research in therapeutic procedures of several types. Dr. Paul G. Quie (1986) presented a definition of **biomedical ethics** at the 1985 annual meeting of the Infectious Diseases Society of America:

Ethics is a formal discipline, a branch of philosophy that seeks to examine the right and wrong of human acts rationally, to discover generalizable principles, to examine the logic of ethical discourse, and to identify assumptions upon which decisions are made. Biomedical Ethics, therefore, is application of ethics to medical decision making.

With this definition in mind, let us attempt to identify principles and guidelines for making decisions about medical and health care practices. In particular, we will look at specific practices or problems created by the application of ethics to the improvement of care and expansion of scientific knowledge, through the involvement of human subjects.

---

*Norma Jean Shira
Associate Professor, Health and Occupational Education, Western Kentucky University, Bowling Green, KY 42101.

Historical Background

You are all familiar with the **Hippocratic Oath**, which states: "I will use treatment to help the sick . . . but never with a view to injury and wrong doing" (Goldfield, 1981). Doctors traditionally take this oath at graduation from medical school, and we have been touched with their concern for the well-being of the patient. Most of us have considered this oath to be an excellent example of medical ethics. In reality, this oath enshrined rules of behavior or etiquette more than rules of moral conduct or ethics.

Medical ethics is a comparatively new field of interest, and reflects problems that have come into existence within the last twenty to thirty years. In earlier days, ethical concerns were not a problem or issue because health care was so very simple: patients either got better or died. Doctors offered remedies that either worked or did not – in either case they may not have been exactly sure why.

It is only in the last thirty years, with medicine and physicians having developed an intensive scientific basis for practice and knowledge, that moral and ethical problems have evolved in health care and medicine. As knowledge increases, the possibilities for medical intervention grow in more and more ways. In addition, medicine has placed such a premium on research that many doctors believe they should be both healers and experimental scientists.

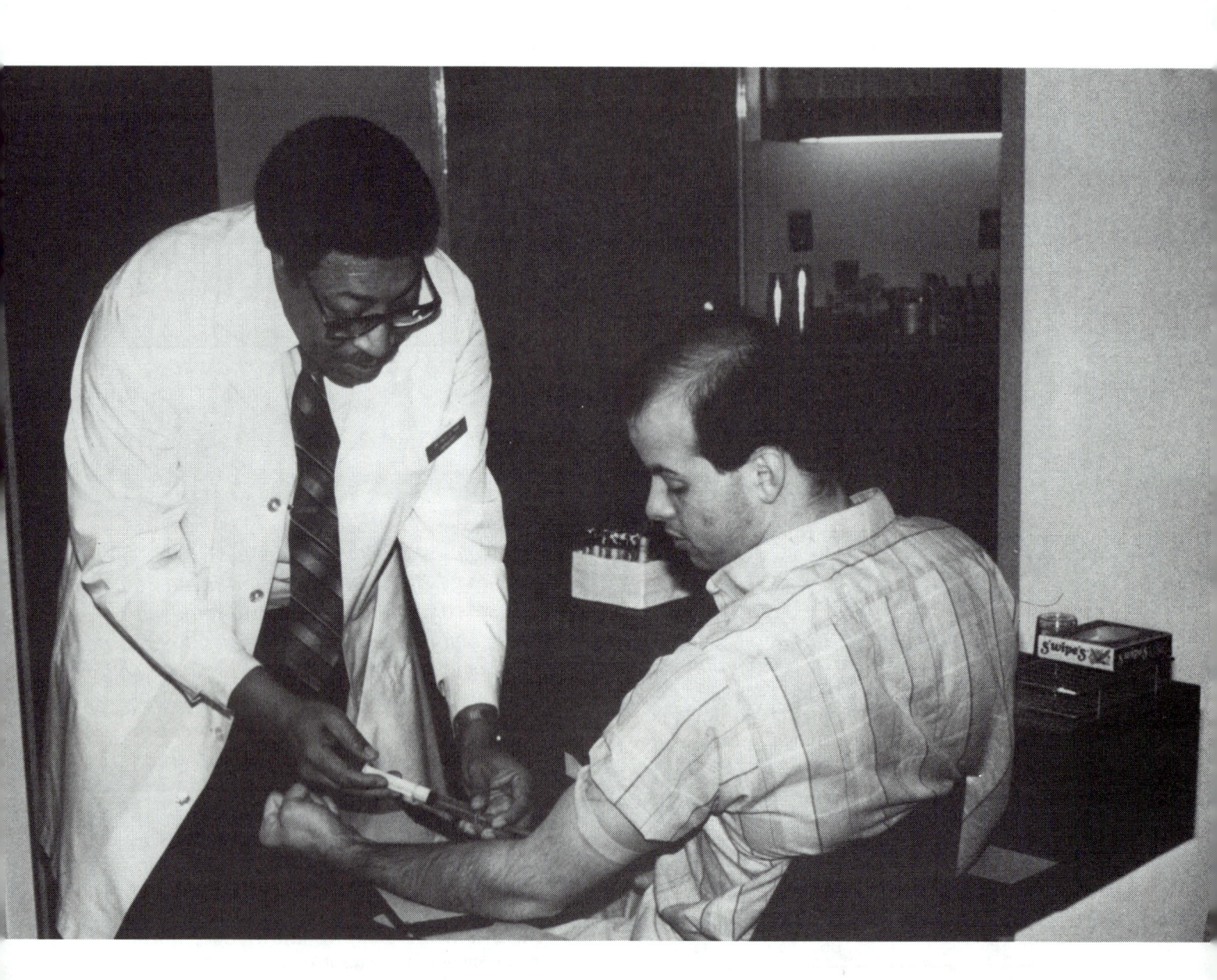

As the need for knowledge intensifies, many health professionals attempt to balance two concerns about research. The first concern deals with the health professional's dedication to the protection of the individual, especially those involved in research as research subjects. The second concern is the recognition of the need for research – and the feeling that it is immoral not to do the necessary research.

This dilemma has grown as scientific knowledge has expanded because medicine is now able to use therapeutic weapons for good, on the one hand, and harm, on the other. Who could have known thirty years ago that the use of X-rays would cause certain types of cancer? Or that the use of detergents and certain synthetics would increase allergies? Or that advances in chemotherapies and other therapeutic procedures would cause the development of a new strain of staphylococcal pathology?

Progress and change of this type is the major reason for continuing a close examination of the relationships between medical science and clinical trials – research involving human subjects. It is out of these inevitable conflicts of knowledge, needs, and interests that important ethical problems and difficult moral dilemmas develop.

Scientific research has produced many benefits to society. It has also created troublesome ethical questions. The general public became concerned with these ethical questions after the Second World War, when the Nuremburg War Crime Trials reported the abuses of human subjects used in biomedical experiments.

The Nuremburg Code, drafted as a result of the war crimes trials, was a set of standards for judging physicians and scientists involved in these experiments on concentration camp prisoners (National Commission for the Protection of Human Subjects, 1978). This code was the basis for the many later codes, or standards, that were developed. These later codes were established to make sure that research involving human subjects would be carried out in an ethical manner. Codes are the rules or guidelines that help research investigators and review committees in their work. Many times these rules do not cover complex situations; they may be in conflict; sometimes they are difficult to interpret, and/or they may not be applicable to the situation. This is when the broader ethical principles and values provide the means of formulating and interpreting new rules.

In any discussion of medical experimentation and research, it is important that we differentiate between biomedical and behavioral research and the practice of accepted therapy. This distinction is necessary in order to identify the activities that should be reviewed for the protection of human subjects in research.

The term **practice** should refer to those interventions that are for the enhancement of the well-being of the patient or client and have a reasonable amount of success attached to them. **Medical or behavioral practice** should provide diagnosis, preventive treatment, or therapy to specific individuals.

The term **research** refers to an activity that is designed to test a hypothesis, permit conclusions to be drawn, and develop or contribute to knowledge. Research should be described by a formal statement setting forth an objective and a clearly stated procedure for achieving that objective.

Research and practice may be carried on at the same time, if the research is designed to evaluate the safety or efficacy of a specific therapy. If the activity identified has an element of research, it should be reviewed for the protection of human subjects.

Protection of Human Subjects

According to a report by the National Commission for the Protection of Human Subjects of Biomedical and Behavioral Research (1978), three principles are the most relevant to research involving human subjects. Although there may be other relevant principles, these three principles are comprehensive and stated in generalizations that are helpful to scientists, subjects, reviewers, and interested citizens. These principles and generalizations do not resolve ethical problems but do provide the framework for analysis of the problem. The three basic principles are:

- respect for persons
- beneficence
- justice

Respect for persons covers two basic ethical convictions:

- that an individual should be treated as an autonomous (independent/self-governing) agent.
- that persons with diminished autonomy should be protected.

An individual is considered to be autonomous when he or she is capable of determining personal goals and making decisions concerning these goals. However, not everyone is capable of self-determination. Respect for the immature and incapacitated requires that we protect them as they mature or remain incapacitated. The extent of protection given should depend on the risk of harm and the likelihood of benefits.

The concept of **beneficence** involves securing or improving the client's well-being. The term is often interpreted to cover acts of kindness or charity that go beyond strict obligation. Two general rules to use with beneficent actions are:

- Do not harm.
- Maximize possible benefits and minimize possible harms.

A difficult question/problem occurs when the research presents more than minimal risk without immediate direct benefit to the subjects involved.

The concept of **justice** involves the sense of "fairness in distribution" or "what is deserved." Another way of interpreting the principle of justice is that equals ought to be treated equally. In what respects should people be treated equally? Based on societal practices, several plans or guidelines have been accepted as equitable ways of distributing burdens and benefits. These include:

- to each an equal share
- to each according to need
- to each according to effort
- to each according to societal contribution
- to each according to merit.

Only recently have these questions become associated with scientific research. During the early years of scientific research involving human subjects, the selection of subjects, or the burden of risk for serving as a subject, fell largely on the poor ward patients, whereas the benefits of the improved care flowed to private patients. The concept of justice comes in when one tries to determine if subjects are being selected because of their availability, their institutionalized and compromised position, or their manipulability – rather than for reasons related to research.

The principles of autonomy (respect for persons), beneficence (risk and benefits), and justice (equal treatment or selection), as defined by the Belmont Report (National Commission for the Protection of Human Subjects, 1978), have been applied through the practices of informed consent, special considerations for certain groups, and randomized clinical trials. These practices have been combined to form guidelines for solutions and analysis of problems related to biomedical research.

Guidelines for Biomedical Research

There can be no doubt about the rapid increase in knowledge, and if there is to be a similar improvement in treatment and quality of life, there is a need for well-designed research. Research of this type requires trials

---

Gas Station Robbery

While robbing a gas station, a young man is shot. Following hospitalization, he is tried, convicted, and sentenced to jail. Six months later he is found to have contracted AIDS. Investigation shows that the blood transfusion he received while hospitalized apparently was the source.

A pharmaceutical company is offering inmates the opportunity to participate in a research program. As is usually the case with drug experimentation, participants will get a special diet, a private room, and increased visiting privileges.

Should this person be allowed to participate? Why?

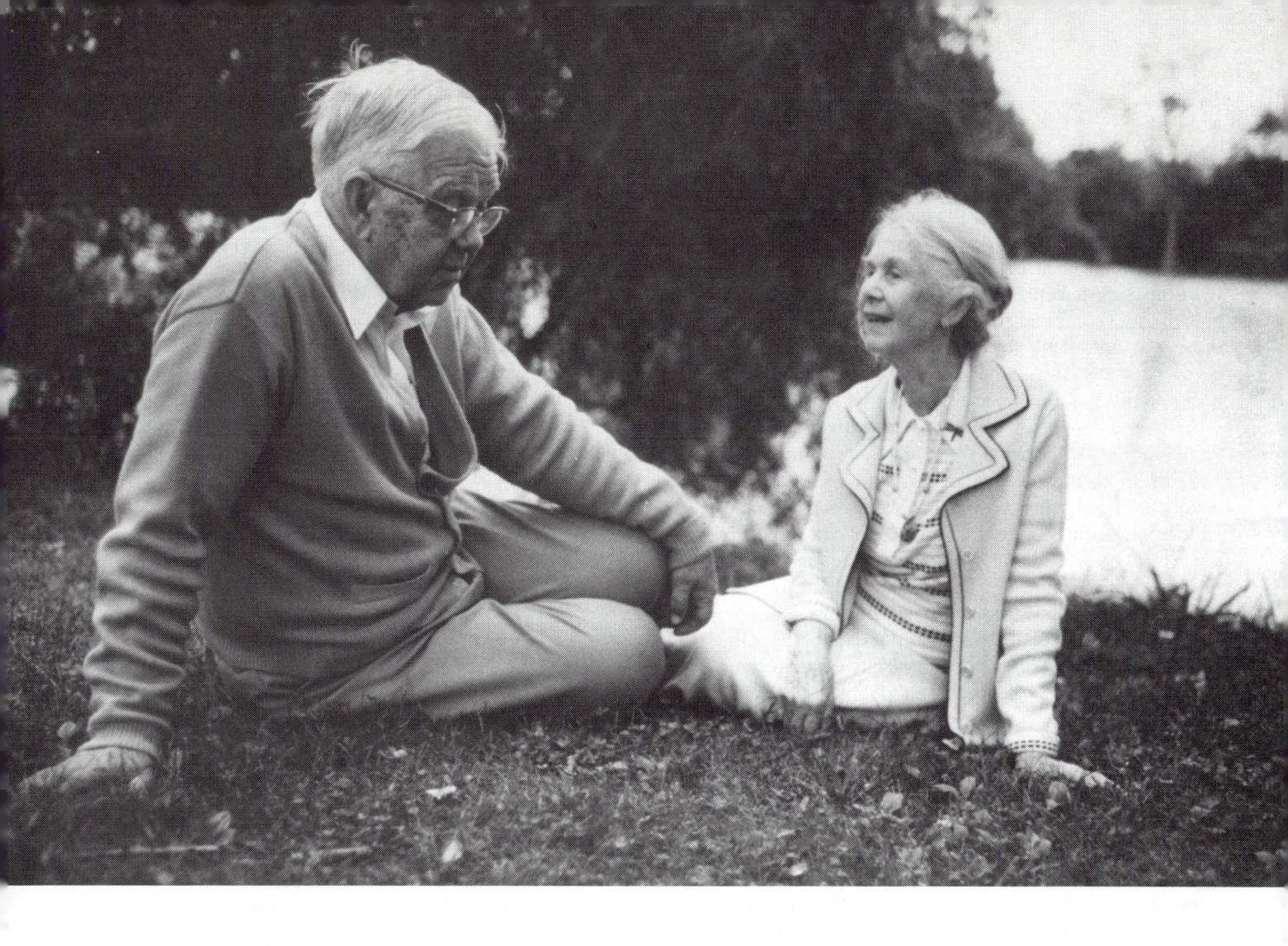

for new drugs and treatments, as well as investigations that may not produce direct benefit to the volunteer undergoing this study.

If we accept the need for research, many ethical problems need to be discussed, and the following ethical guidelines should be included.

Standards of Research

Each research project should have a clearly defined, reasonably attainable objective, and the research design and methods should be appropriate to achieve that objective.

Do Certain Groups Require Special Ethical Consideration?

Much has been written about the problems of research on specific groups, such as children or prisoners, and the extra safeguards suggested for their protection. Recent issues relating to the use of the elderly in research show that this specific group may be penalized and/or hurt more than some of the other groups. The elderly may be a desirable group to use in research for several reasons:

- People are living longer, and research is needed on those conditions that cause health and social problems.

- The elderly in hospitals and nursing homes provide a stable population for monitoring and controlling activities, drug therapy, and medical conditions.

- The institutionalized elderly may acquiesce to research participation rather than consent (promise of reward or better care – similar to the situation with prisoners in jail).

- The elderly patient may feel that "you have helped me, so I will take part in your research."

For a given group, special considerations must be given to maintain autonomy, beneficence, and justice.

The Problem of Consent

In any research involving human subjects, this is a real problem. In the case of the elderly, many may have special needs, but most may be able to make reasonable decisions about their care and can handle most of their own finances. It is possible for many, from this elderly group, to give consent for participation in research. But those who are unable to make reasoned decisions – the confused and demented – present problems and need to be considered as a special group. It is legally wrong to interfere or intervene physically with another person without his or her consent.

In addition, the concept of **consent** means full or adequate consent. Just how much should the volunteer and the physicians be told about the specific details of the research? The idea of "full disclosure" needed for fully informed consent may produce confusion and anxiety in the volunteer. Many times the physician may withhold harmful or distressing information from the patient to maintain the emotional stability of the patient. The physician can legally withhold information when it is deemed in the best interest of the patient.

The problem of consent, especially in the elderly and other special groups, may be dependent on the level of mental competence of the individual. There are those who may be able to handle their day-to-day decisions and cope with financial affairs, but who may not understand the requirements of a research procedure. Consent in this situation should include a determination of competence and the extent to which the individual understands the research procedure.

The consent form, in itself, does not guarantee that explanations and understandings are adequate. The form should list in understandable, easily read language, the following:

* purposes of the research
* procedures involved
* risks and benefits to the volunteer
* freedom to withdraw from the research
* freedom to ask questions about research and/or the voluntary involvement

The Use of Randomized Clinical Trials

When a new treatment is being assessed and compared with an existing or established treatment, **randomized clinical trials** are used. The purpose is to find out if one treatment is better than another. The research volunteer will receive a known good treatment or one that may be better. The ethics in this situation deals with the determination of one treatment over another. Many health professionals believe that the use of randomized clinical trials verges on the unethical. They offer the following arguments against clinical experimentation:

* It is incompatible with good clinical care.
* It is unacceptable to the patient.
* It is unrealistic.
* The results are not used.
* It has no scientific merit or value.
* It can be very expensive.

Another area of controversy with randomized clinical trials relates to the use of **placebos** (an inert substance made to appear like a drug being tested). Many believe that the use of placebos will deny treatment to a patient who needs it. Ethical consideration must be given to the use of placebos when there is no known effective treatment, and when determining whether the patient should have "full disclosure" about the research.

To be of value, all clinical trials must be well designed, with clearly stated and attainable objectives; and with the selection of patients and controls being made very carefully.

Monitoring Research

All committees responsible for the monitoring or review of research involving human subjects have outstanding problems. The review monitors are responsible for determining whether the researcher obtained consent correctly, followed the line of research, had any ethical problems or difficulties, and whether the committees can learn or gain from these difficulties.

Concerns Related to Biomedical Ethics

Biomedical ethics is an appropriate topic for health practitioners and educators, since we are responsible for helping with decision making about the ethics of medical and health care practice. Unfortunately, there are no real "answers" in these ethical discussions, but this does not detract from their importance. Ethical questions are particularly important because many of the new medical procedures are highly technical, scarce, and costly, and hence cannot be practiced on everyone in need; because as health professionals we feel a duty to provide the best care to patients; and because certain types of inherent restrictions are a reality in health care and service.

At the present time, the ethical and moral questions that occur most frequently for health professionals and researchers include the following topics (Goldfield, 1981):

- **Money versus life**. Who pays for the best care? Can we afford to keep people alive through high technology? Is it the right of every human being to have the world's best medical care at any cost?

- **Doctor versus patient.** Are all patients capable of giving informed consent? According to the decisions of the Supreme Court, every human being of sound mind has a right to determine what shall be done with his or her own body. But should that right extend to the mentally ill, elderly, children, or other special groups?

- **Life versus life.** When there is a chance to save a transplantable organ, should a dying patient's final minutes be sacrificed so that someone else might live? Who should have my heart? Should mechanical life support measures be stopped, and an operation performed, or do you wait for the heart to stop?

- **Government versus the public.** Do we have the right to choose our own medical treatments even though the treatment may be unorthodox? Can a family or patient reject an accepted but extremely painful treatment in favor of another, newer or unapproved, treatment of their choice? How does this affect the concept of informed consent for the special groups – children and/or incompetent?

- **Science versus public**. Does the public have the right to know all about the latest medical research – even if that information might be confusing, frightening, incomplete, or even dangerous? How much should the researcher reveal to the public through the media?

- **Government versus science.** Scientific research can, and perhaps will, present humanity with overwhelming dangers. Should the government have the power to step in? Should a DNA machine, when perfected, be banned?

The issues of Government versus the Public, Science versus the Public, and Government versus Science are perhaps best exemplified by some of the dilemmas of today's society.

The Federal Government, because of laws and regulations for testing and evaluation, may restrict the use of new treatments and drugs developed in foreign countries. Many times only the benefits of the new practices may be described, and the difficulties and side effects may not be discussed publicly. This provides incomplete information to those concerned with decisions about general use. The Government may then become involved with the "protection of the populus" concept and evoke the federal laws for control.

The dilemmas are demonstrated by the laetrile controversy, the controversy about research on the use of cannabis for the relief of pain in glaucoma and chemotherapy and nausea in cancer, the current controversy in the research and development of drugs and treatments for persons with AIDS, the controversy about the multihandicapped and genetically deformed infants such as Baby Doe, and the controversies about the choice of treatment for terminally ill children when accepted treatment is against the religious beliefs of the family.

Summary

You need to remember that the way in which medical ethics makes its most valuable contribution is not by offering to solve specific problems to the satisfaction of all, but by providing us with an increased awareness that these concerns or problems have occurred in our society and must be taken seriously. Eventually we may find answers by observing the actions of teachers and peers we respect, and by behaving in a similar manner. If and when new and more sensitive attitudes become part of our society, we may not need to discuss these topics further. Until that time, we must be diligent in our attention and thoughts about these questions.

Cited References

Goldfield, June (1981, October). The toughest moral questions in medicine. *Health*, the Magazine for Total Well-Being, 13 (9): 40-50.

National Commission for the Protection of Human Subjects of Biomedical and Behavioral Research (1978). *The Belmont Report: ethical principles and guidelines for the protection of human subjects of research*. Washington, D.C. Government Printing Office, DHEW Publication No. (OS) 78-0012).

Quie, Paul G. (1986, March). Health care economics and biomedical ethics. *Journal of Infectious Diseases*, 153 (3): 385-389.

Additional Bibliography

Bolotin, Carol. (1985, June). Drug as HERO. *Science*, 68-71.

Denham, Michael. (1984, January 18). Ethics of research. *Nursing Mirror*, 158: (1): 36-38.

Drummond, Rennie, M.D. (1982, April 17). Informed consent by well-nigh abject adults. Editorial. *New England Journal of Medicine*, 302 (16): 917-18.

Hayflick, Leonard. (1985). Future directions in aging research. *Basic Life Sciences*, 35: 447-60.

Krauthammer, Charles. (1981, December 9). The ethics of human experimentation. *The New Republic*, 16-19.

Levine, Robert J. (1986, March/April). Medical science, the clinical trial and society. *Hastings Center Report*, 3 (2): 19-21.

Masson, Alison, and Rubin, Paul H. (1985, August 22). Matching prescription drugs and consumers – the benefits of direct advertising. Sounding board. *New England Journal of Medicine*, 313 (8): 513-15.

Moran, Michael G., and Thompson, Troy L., II. (1986, March). The use of psychotropic drugs in geriatric patients. *Medical Times, 114 (3): 33-38.*

Nelson, Harry. (1986, March 6). Patients pay to be part of cancer tests. *Los Angeles Times,* San Diego County, California.

Oberst, Marilyn T. (1985, November-December). Another look at informed consent, point/counterpoint. *Nursing Outlook*, 33 (6) 294-95.

Ratsan, Richard Martyn (1981). The experiment that wasn't: a case report in clinical geriatric research. *The Gerontologist*, 21 (3): 297-302.

Schafer, Arthur. (1982, September 16). The ethics of the randomized clinical trial. *New England Journal of Medicine*, 307: 320-24.

Schneider, E. L. (1985). Aging research: challenge of the twenty-first century. *Basic Life Sciences*. 35: 1-11.

Shaffer, Mary K., and Pfeiffer, Isobell L. (1986, January). Nursing research and patient's rights. *American Journal of Nursing*, 23-24.

Veatch, Robert M., and Sallitto, Sharmon (1973, June). Human experimentation, the ethical questions persist. *Hastings Center Report*, 3 (3): 22-24.

Mark and Experimental Drugs

Mark is a thirteen-year-old epileptic whose seizures cannot be controlled by conventional medication. His father is a successful trial lawyer who has one dream, that Mark will join his law firm. Obviously, if Mark's condition should continue, it will keep him from such a career.

The family doctor has learned about a new experimental drug which he thinks will control Mark's seizures appreciably better. However, this drug has a number of possible side effects and can only be obtained in Europe, still needing approval by the Food and Drug Administration in this country. The two known side effects of concern are gynecomastic enlargement (swelling of the breasts) and a high pitch to the voice. Long-term effects are not yet established because of the newness of the drug.

Mark's parents have been told about the new drug therapy, and they share the information with Mark, who is concerned about his body image, having a high voice, and what his friends will say. He doesn't have a lot of friends and often feels lonely. He wonders whether he will lose those friends he has and if all the other students at school will tease him.

The doctor recommends counseling and family therapy before consenting to this drug therapy and is somewhat cautious about the treatment. Mark's parents appear to be eager for him to use the drug, whereas Mark refuses to talk about the therapy.

- Are the possible side effects regarded with equal importance by Mark and his family?
- If something were to go wrong at some later time, is it possible for Mark to sue the doctor who used the experimental drug on him?
- Suppose Mark's parents decide to go ahead with the treatment. Does Mark have any recourse?
- Could Mark sue his parents at a later time if they insist that he take the treatment, considering that they were only trying to improve the quality of his life?
- Suppose Mark agrees to undergo the treatment, and he does get enlarged breasts. Should the change be as important to him as the control over his epileptic seizures that he gets from the new medicine?
- Are people taking an unnecessary chance using a new drug therapy before it is fully checked for immediate and long-term actions?
- Should people use drugs that are accepted in other countries but not in the United States?
- If Mark were to take the medication and get enlarged breasts, should the school excuse him from taking physical education, where this change might be noticed?
- Should Mark be pressured to undergo this experimental therapy, considering he is a minor?
- What action might be taken to ensure that the parents are not considering the therapy because of a feeling of embarrassment at Mark's seizures or some feeling of guilt?
- Suppose the researchers have a time frame that does not allow Mark to undergo psychological evaluation and family counseling. Should he still take the drug therapy?
- Considering that there might be benefits to be derived from the research, what risk should be permitted?
- Frequently experimental drug therapy carries with it an expectation that the patient will agree to be interviewed at the conclusion of the experimentation. Should Mark have to be interviewed if he is still a minor?
- Should he be interviewed because of the nature of the side effects and the type of problem that he has?
- Suppose the news media find out about the experimentation and want information. If Mark refuses to discuss it, should the doctor conducting the study tell about Mark?

10

Medicine's Chaos: The Terminally Ill

Margaret Snell*

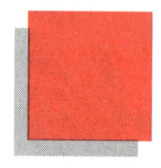

Objectives

After reading this chapter you should be able to:
- Define the terms listed in the beginning of this chapter.
- Discuss some of the attitudes about death and dying common to nomadic and agricultural societies.
- Describe the ancient Greek and Roman beliefs about death and dying, and compare them with Judeo-Christian beliefs.
- Trace the development of interest in euthanasia in this century.
- Understand the function of ethics committees and living wills.
- Describe the general positions held by the major faiths regarding euthanasia.
- Discuss some landmark cases involving active and passive euthanasia.
- Describe, in general terms, international practices regarding euthanasia.
- Summarize the current status of euthanasia in the United States.

Terms and Definitions

Euthanasia. The original meaning was an "easy death"; however, in modern usage it means termination of a life associated with suffering.

Active euthanasia. A process in which some means is used, such as injecting a lethal dose of a chemical, to end the life of a terminally ill person rapidly and in comfort, as opposed to allowing life to end slowly as a result of the condition.

Passive euthanasia. Care that is limited to caring for a person's physical needs, including assistance in breathing and nutritional feeding; nothing else is done to prolong life.

Irreversible coma. A condition in which the person is in a coma and appears to be sleeping, though there is no possibility of the person returning to wellness.

Persistent vegetative state. A nonreversible condition of extensive brain damage in which the individual may seem to respond to certain stimuli and to awake at times, though neither is the case.

Terminal illness. An irreversible medical condition that will result in death.

Introduction

People in every society share a concern about how life may be ended. They have specific rules about this, although these rules may vary from one society to another because people place different values on life.

Our society is no exception. We used to have guidelines on how a person might die. Today, medical care technology has evolved in sophistication and complexity to the point that people can be kept alive almost indefinitely. These advances have led to changes in the rules about how to keep a person alive, but no new rules have evolved regarding how a person may die.

People are becoming aware that new guidelines are needed, and they are mandating that they be established and practiced. The process of defining and agreeing to new rules, however, is creating considerable confusion and disagreement; some might even say chaos. To understand what is happening, it is worthwhile to be informed about the practices of the past and the influences in practice at this time. This chapter discusses how people in other societies allowed life to be ended and provides an overview of some of the influences that have an impact on how life might be terminated in our society.

*Margaret Snell
Associate Professor and Director, Health Care Education, Chair, Education Department, Cook College
Rutgers University, New Brunswick, NJ 08903

Nomadic and Agricultural Tribes

In the nomadic and agricultural societies that were common before the industrial revolution, attitudes about death and dying were related to age. If a person did not or could not contribute to the survival of the group, his or her death was not considered important.

Children were regarded with mixed emotions. If times were hard, children were not welcomed regardless of how much people wanted to have a child. If one were born, it meant another mouth to feed. Most preindustrial societies had ways to abort an unwanted pregnancy, and the practice was widespread (Devereux, 1955). Indeed, when food was short, people showed little concern when a young child died or a pregnancy was lost.

People were more upset when an adult died. It was even considered a major crisis in some instances, particularly when the group's survival could be compromised. The loss of a hunter or a very strong person was felt by the entire group.

Adults lived a very hazardous life in most early societies, with few of them reaching old age. Among the hazards and problems were starvation, accidents, disease, environmental problems, and, depending on the culture, possibly the need to migrate. Enemy attacks also were a constant threat. Life could end suddenly and violently. It was an achievement to live to middle age. Those who lived beyond it were weakened by disease and the problems of old age. They were unable to hunt or to tend to the crops. Sometimes they even threatened the group's survival by eating food that was in short supply.

Some societies honored old age. The Murgin of Australia showed old people great respect (Warner,

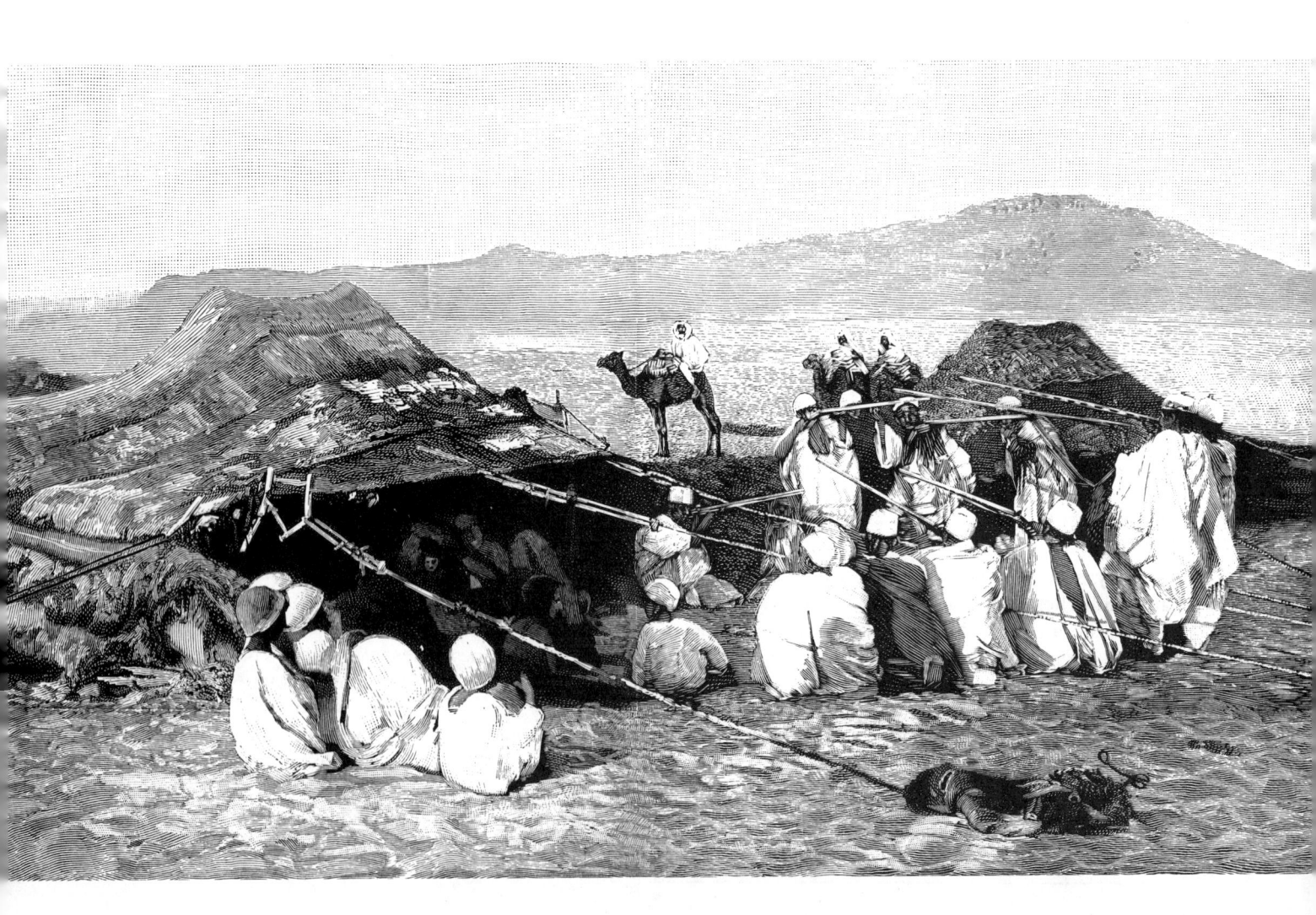

1937). The elderly knew the history and folklore of the tribe. Because of that, they were regarded as very important people in the tribe. Their advice was asked and followed, their death regarded as a tragedy.

But not all agricultural cultures respected or even wanted old people. In describing the lifestyle of the Hopi Indian, Kennard (1937) said that people were expected to die when they got old and were no longer productive. He found that the older people got, the less respect they received. Initially they were treated with indifference and excluded from social and religious activities. After a time they were neglected, and some were even treated cruelly. In some instances people were told that they were taking too long to die. The old and even the sick were expected to wander away from the group to die, either by starvation or from exposure.

The elderly who lived in cultures honoring old age made preparations for their death (Simmons, 1970). When the time came to die, they were surrounded by their family and their friends. Sometimes they stopped eating, and at times they took other measures. Regardless of how much they were loved and admired, they were never encouraged to prolong their life.

The attitude of encouraging or at least not discouraging death was common in agricultural and early cultures and particularly true of nomadic tribes. When it came time to migrate, it was not uncommon for some of the elderly to be left behind (Warner, 1937). Survival was a very serious business in those early times, and emotions were ruled by necessity. Some tribes even killed the sick, infirm, and elderly when group survival depended on it.

Greek-Roman Antiquity and Judeo-Christian Beliefs

The prevailing attitude toward dying in ancient Greece and Rome was that people had the right to end their own life (Gruman, 1978). They could even get help to do so. At times a person might even be respected for taking his own life, as in the case of Socrates when he drank hemlock. The term **euthanasia**, meaning easy death, comes from this period.

In Sparta a father was required by law to submit his newborn child to a council for examination (Ostheimer and Ostheimer, 1976). If the child was male and strong, he was given a piece of land. Children who were mentally or physically weak were thrown into a hole in the ground to die. Such children were considered a burden to the state, and the parents were not allowed to keep them.

Until the start of the seventeenth century, people tolerated individuals who chose to end their life (Gruman, 1978). Early in that century, however, medical knowledge developed to the point that physicians began to recognize that certain actions seemed to allow someone to die, perhaps even to hasten a person's death. They began to speak about these actions as euthanasia. Other activities were recognized as prolonging life. Those came to be regarded as **life support activities.**

Controversy developed regarding how much should be done to ward off death, who had responsibility for a person's death, whether death was voluntary, and whether death resulted from certain actions (Gruman, 1978). Judeo-Christian beliefs became the basis of these arguments. The same concerns are still being discussed today.

Eastern Cultures: A Different Perspective

Eastern societies have a different perspective on old age and death than do other societies. Reynolds (1961) identified three distinct traditions within the eastern societies: the Sinitic tradition, including Confucian and Taoist influences; the Vedic-Hindu tradition; and the Buddhist tradition.

Sinitic tradition is oriented to the world as we know it. A person is expected to live a careful existence designed to preserve his or her body and to seek long life. By comparison, the Vedic-Hindu tradition is more fatalistic toward death. A current life reflects how someone lived in a previous one. People are concerned with trying to live as well as possible to achieve karma. Buddhism is concerned with rebirth, and there is a strong emphasis to live life as well as possible and to respect life in general.

Overview of Euthanasia in the Twentieth Century

In the beginning of this century, little was written that supported euthanasia, though by the thirties interest started to build for dying with dignity (Oden, 1976). Euthanasia societies were established both in the United States and in England, and legislation was suggested. World War II cooled enthusiasm for euthanasia, however, in large part because of Hitler's disposal of those people he considered unfit to live.

After the war, interest in euthanasia revived. For the first time medical and legal journals began printing right-to-die articles. The phenomenal growth of lifesaving technology also created major ethical problems, and euthanasia was thrust into the limelight. Legislation supporting it was introduced in the United States and in Europe (Veatch, 1978).

Nebraska was the first state to consider an euthanasia bill in 1937. The bill was not passed, nor were similar bills in Idaho in 1969, Florida in 1970, West Virginia in 1972, and Oregon in 1973. Interest in euthanasia legislation continued, however.

Until recently people who had severe congenital abnormalities or those who were accidentally reduced to a vegetative state died quickly. People who developed incurable illnesses also died relatively fast. This happened because medical practitioners lacked the knowledge and the means to continue life. The sophisticated technology of today was still to be developed.

Advances over the last decade or so are generally acknowledged to have exceeded all medical progress in the past hundred years. These advances in medical technology have occurred with increasing frequency and show no sign of stopping. As a result, the unwritten differentiation between what is ordinary care and extraordinary care has become obscured. Pacemakers, hemodialysis, and respirators are no longer considered exotic types of health care. Rather, they are fast becoming aspects of routine care. More and more frequently people are being snatched back from death.

Why?

Technology is creating many questions, not about saving lives, but about when it is appropriate to let a life go. Tifft (1983) provides a provocative example. An elderly dying patient was revived from death. He was unable to speak but wrote the following message to the doctor, "Why did you do this?"

The Confusion about Terminology

Death is one word most people know. If they do not know it as children, they do by the time they reach adulthood. The word used to mean the cessation of spontaneous respiration and heartbeat. This was determined by listening for a heartbeat with a stethoscope and attempting to locate a pulse. When they were not found, it meant that the person was no longer living. Determining whether someone was dead was not a great problem. Everyone knew that when someone stopped breathing, the person was dead.

No longer can **death** be so easily defined. Barnard (1980) calls attention to the various kinds of death that have to be considered. Physicians speak about **brain death, biological death,** and **cellular death,** signifying the different parts of the body that are dead. These various terms signal that death is considered a process. No longer is a dying person thought to be alive one minute and dead the next. In some instances it is even possible for someone to be somewhere between the two, in what is commonly known as a **vegetative state**, neither alive nor dead.

A terminal illness is defined by the Los Angeles County Medical Association ("Principles and Guidelines," 1985) as an irreversible medical condition that will cause the patient's death in a time period from weeks to months, but no longer than a year. Some people might ask about the person who is dying but does not do so within the twelve-month deadline. Does that person have a terminal illness or not? Despite their shortcomings, definitions are necessary and useful; this one is similar to those used by other medical associations.

People tend to be confused by what is meant by an irreversible coma and a persistent vegetative state. An **irreversible coma** typically means that a person survives for a limited period even through life support systems are used. Patients in a coma do not open their eyes, and appear to be asleep. People in a **persistent vegetative state** may be maintained for months or even

Mrs. Simone Wishing to Die

Mrs. Simone's husband has been dead for about a year when Maria, her daughter, gets married. Soon after that, Maria's husband is transferred to another part of the country, some distance away. Mrs. Simone feels very badly about Maria getting married, and when she hears that her daughter will be moving away she cries and becomes very depressed. Maria says that she will come home on vacation to see her mother and that her mother will, of course, come to visit her. Nevertheless, Mrs. Simone remains very upset.

About a month after her daughter moves, Mrs. Simone gets a cold which gets progressively worse. She tells her friends and neighbors that they are not to inform her daughter, that "she will get even with them for moving away and leaving her." They promise not to tell anyone.

A week or so later Mrs. Simone starts to wheeze. She has an elevated temperature and must be hospitalized. Mrs. Simone refuses to eat. When pressured, she only picks at her food. She continues to be depressed, but refuses to have her daughter contacted. The doctor finds that she has a heart condition and starts to medicate her for that. Mrs. Simone refuses to take her heart medicine, and when a nurse insists, she pretends she has taken it and then throws the pill away.

The doctor then sends her to a nursing home. Mrs. Simone agrees to go so long as her daughter isn't told. Once there, however, she again refuses to take her medication and cannot be coaxed to eat. Within a few days she contracts pneumonia and pulmonary edema. Her heart condition becomes progressively worse. When the doctor comes to see her, she says that she wants to die; she has nothing to live for. She refuses all food and medication. A nasogastric feeding tube is inserted, but Mrs. Simone removes the tube and demands to be allowed to die. She says that it is her right to refuse treatment, and she again demands that her daughter not be informed. She goes on to say that she will continue to write to her daughter what she wants her to know and that it is no one else's business.

What should be done and why?

years. People who are in a persistent vegetative state may seem to respond to certain stimuli, may appear to be awake at times and asleep at other times. This confusion also makes decision making regarding care very difficult.

Euthanasia is derived from the Greeks, with **Eu** meaning well or easy and **thanatos** meaning death. The meaning at that time was a painless, happy death. Modern usage has modified this word to mean an act involving a painless death or a termination of suffering.

Euthanasia may be classified as active, passive, voluntary, involuntary, voluntary active, voluntary passive, involuntary passive, or involuntary active. The following definitions were used in the House of Delegates of the American Medical Association on December 4, 1973 (Steinbock, 1980), and will give a sense of what the various terms mean. **Voluntary euthanasia** and **active euthanasia** usually mean the person decides to end his or her own suffering. **Passive euthanasia** involves others making that decision. It also can mean that nature is allowed to take its course. Passive euthanasia involves the withholding or omitting of extraordinary treatment that might extend life. Active euthanasia can be either voluntary (with the patient's consent) or involuntary (without the patient's consent).

The distinction between the types of euthanasia is essential in medical ethics. Withholding treatment and allowing a patient to die are considered permissible in some cases. It is against the law to take any direct action to kill a person. Most physicians also consider it morally wrong to take any direct action designed to kill a patient regardless of the circumstances.

Living Wills and Ethics Committees

Most people do not die unexpectedly. According to Tifft (1983) approximately 80 percent of people currently die in a hospital or nursing home. Modern technology has given physicians some major weapons to use in taking care of patients. It also has provided a major dilemma. Physicians are faced with the problem of imposing life on people who are suffering. Should they prolong this suffering? Do they have an option to do otherwise?

Consider the case of Eli Kahn, who was admitted to the hospital when he was seventy-eight. He described himself as a broken down engine and asked to be allowed to die with dignity. In spite of his wishes, medical treatment was instituted, and he was connected to a mechanical respirator. During the night he managed to turn off the machine. Before he died, he wrote the following message to his physician, "Death is not the enemy, doctor, inhumanity is." (Barnard, 1980, p. 8).

Living wills assist physicians in determining what type of care to provide to patients. In essence a living will means that a person decides and documents the nature and extent of medical care he or she wishes to receive in the event that circumstances or illness should render that person incapable of making a decision. These directions are given while the person is competent and in good health and are conveyed to family and friends. When people do not formalize their wishes, problems can occur at a later time.

Jackson and Youngner (1979) specify that disease, pain, and drugs plus a variety of other conditions alter a patient's ability to make decisions regarding the nature and degree of care that should be provided. The most important consideration is the competence of the patient at the time a decision must be made. In terminal illnesses some people believe that a patient's decision-making ability progressively decreases. Thus living wills provide an important basis for determining what the patient would like to have done.

California passed the first law describing what an adult person may direct the physician to do – follow life-sustaining procedures or withhold or withdraw them – in the event of a terminal condition (Veatch, 1978). Thirty-nine states now have living will statutes. According to Mehling (1986), all states except North Dakota have had bills before them.

In spite of directives in advance from a patient with a terminal illness, many physicians have a fear of legal liability if their care even hints at euthanasia. Also complicating the issue of whether to continue aggressive treatment are the physician's personal values and unconscious motivations. Making a decision to suspend treatment can be as traumatic for the physician as for the patient's family.

A critical issue involving care of a terminally ill patient is the patient's competency. Is the person able to be involved in decision making? When a person is found to be incompetent and there is no living will, the physician must depend on the family and a long-standing relationship with the patient to determine what type of care to give. When the family does not agree with what a patient has requested or cannot agree among themselves, the doctor is faced with a real dilemma.

Another consideration is that terminally ill people often are cared for by physicians who do not have any long-standing relationship with them. A specialist or member of the house staff usually has no knowledge about what a patient would have wanted. When this bad situation is made worse by a family that cannot agree, physicians need assistance. An ethics committee is one answer.

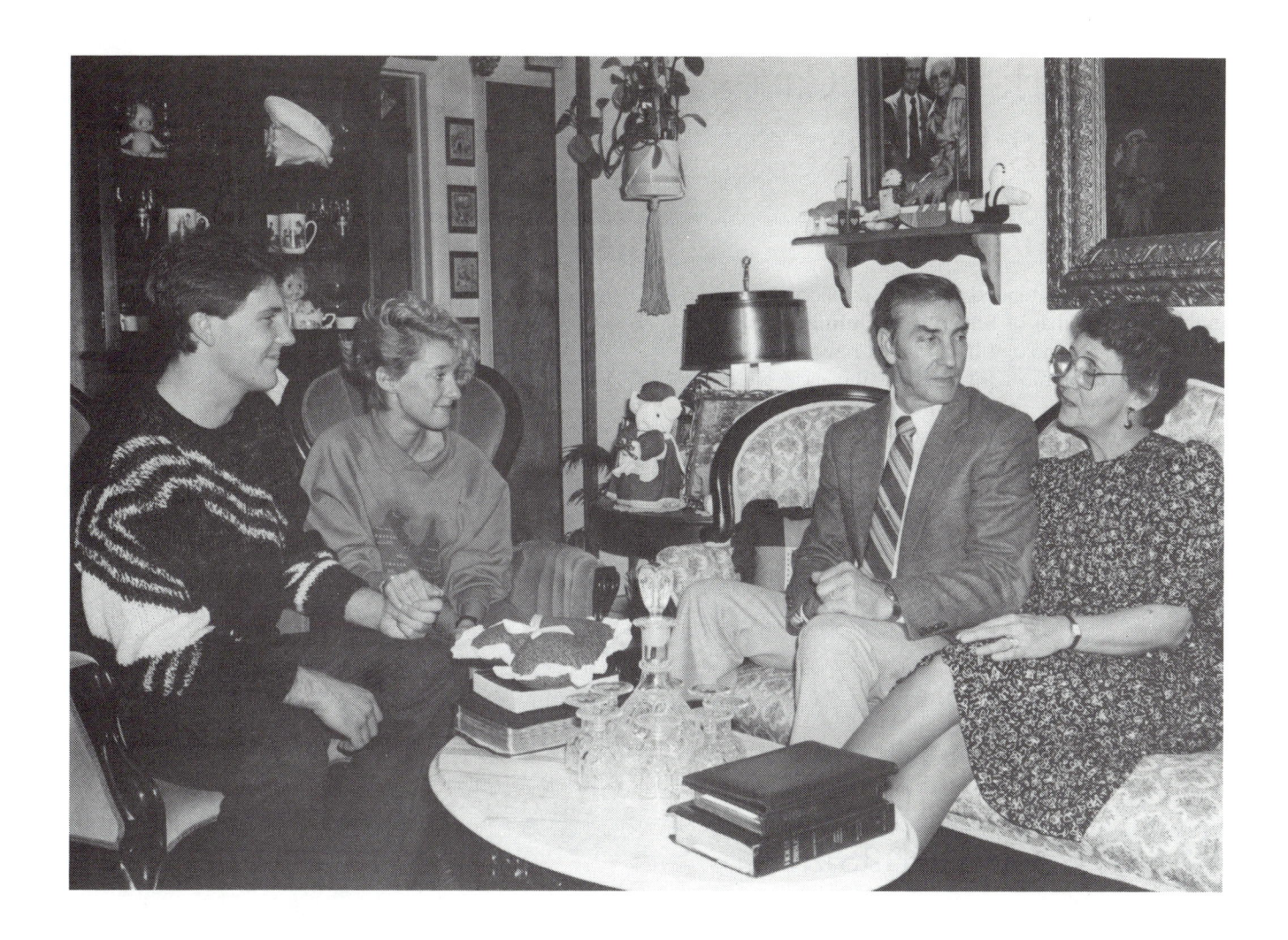

An **ethics committee** is a relatively new way of trying to identify the best action to take in a particular situation. These committees are composed of such individuals as physicians, administrators, lawyers, and representatives of the clergy. Serving in an advisory capacity, they offer guidance to physicians and members of the family.

A 1976 poll by the American Medical Association (Stein, 1978) revealed that 71 percent of the physicians surveyed indicated they asked their patients' wishes about the type of care they wished to receive. Of these, 95 percent said they tried to follow their patient's wishes.

Positions of the Major Faiths

Among the major faiths, there is agreement that it is morally permissible to allow a person to die if therapy will not lead to recovery (Tifft, 1983). It is generally believed that an individual has the responsibility to live as long as he or she can; however, when it becomes apparent that the person is going to die, there seems to be no obligation for the person to prolong life. In terms of resuscitation efforts for a dying patient, Pope Pius XII (1958, p. 394) describes the omission of therapy as "never more than an indirect cause of the cessation of life."

Landmark Court Cases Involving Passive Euthanasia

The case that tended to focus public attention on euthanasia was that of **Karen Ann Quinlan**. It showed that medical technology had created new ethical, legal, and moral dilemmas. Involved in the case were the patient's rights to privacy and the state's interest in preserving life. (See accompanying box).

Other Cases Involving Passive Euthanasia

The case that erased the legal distinction between ventilators and artificial feeding tubes was the **Clair Conroy** case. Conroy was a nursing home resident who was being fed by a nasogastric tube. Her family petitioned the court to remove the feeding tube. They stated that Conroy would not have wanted to be kept alive in that fashion. The court refused the request. An appeal to the New Jersey Supreme Court affirmed the right of the eighty-four-year-old incompetent, terminally ill patient to refuse all medical care (*Right-to-die court decisions*, 1988).

The Conroy decision involved an elderly patient. The court still had to rule on whether a younger patient should continue to receive nourishment. **Nancy Jobes** was a thirty-year-old, healthy woman in her fifth month of pregnancy when she was involved in an automobile accident. Although she was not badly injured, her unborn baby was killed. During an operation to remove the dead fetus, she suffered an acute cardiopulmonary collapse when oxygen was cut off to her brain, and she became brain dead. The family's request to the lower court that artificial sustenance be removed was denied. An appeal was initiated and granted (*Right-to-die decisions*, 1988).

The Case of Karen Ann Quinlan

On April 15, 1975, Karen Ann Quinlan was admitted to a New Jersey hospital. When she was transferred later to Saint Clare's Hospital, she was unconscious and on a respirator. Electroencephalogram (EEG) findings (measuring electrical activity of her brain) were abnormal, but other tests including a brain scan were within normal limits. General medical consensus was that Quinlan was comatose. Her reflexes were on a primitive level. She was nourished by a nasogastric tube and was assisted in breathing by a respirator. She was regarded as being in a persistent vegetative state (Steinbock, 1980).

Because Quinlan was an adult, her father appealed to the court to make him guardian. He wanted the extraordinary procedures discontinued. The Superior Court denied the request. Other legal procedures followed, and the order was finally granted to discontinue the respirator. Quinlan continued to breathe on her own and to be fed by artificial means. She died on July 11, 1985, after being a coma for ten years (Colen, 1976, Davis, 1984, Quinlan and Quinlan, 1977).

In the preceding cases the health care facility agreed to abide by the physician's (and courts') decision. The following case came about because the hospital did not wish to terminate the artificial feedings (*Right-to-die decisions*, 1988). **Paul Brophy** had been in a vegetative state for two years with no hope for recovery when his family requested that the tube feedings be terminated. The hospital Brophy was in did not wish to discontinue them. The family took the issue to court. Approximately a year later the Massachusetts Supreme Court ruled that if the hospital did not want to discontinue the feedings, it had to allow Mr. Brophy to be transferred to another one that would honor the family's wish. Brophy lived eight days once the feedings were stopped.

Whereas Brophy was permanently unconscious, a **Mrs. Raquenna** was alert and aware of what was going on. She had amyotrophic lateral sclerosis (Lou Gehrig's disease) and specifically requested that no feeding devices be used. She was asked to leave the hospital if she did not wish to have tube feedings. Raquenna did not wish to do so. She had an emotional attachment to the staff. She was paralyzed, on a respirator, and deteriorating rapidly. She wanted to stay where she was. The New Jersey Superior Court overruled the hospital and supported her wish. Raquenna was allowed to stop her feedings and to remain at the hospital where she felt she was getting the emotional support that she needed. In essence the court said that hospitals must follow patients' wishes regarding feeding tubes and that emotional support is an essential part of caring for a patient.

The cases cited involve decisions by the court regarding what should be done. Specifically, permission was asked before action was taken. In the case of **Clarence Herbert**, two physicians were charged with murder for discontinuing mechanical ventilation and intravenous feedings. They did not go to court but followed the wishes of the family. This was the first case in which criminal charges were raised (Lo, 1984). The charges were not brought by the family but by a health care practitioner.

Herbert was a fifty-five-year-old security guard who suffered cardiopulmonary arrest during an operation. He never regained consciousness after the operation. His family requested that all machines be removed. Herbert continued to breathe even though the ventilator was removed. Then the family asked that the intravenous fluids be discontinued. After Herbert died, the appellate court examined the circumstances and ruled that murder had not been committed.

The Herbert case (Barber versus Superior Court) has important implications. The court equated discontinuing intravenous feeding with the removal of a respirator or any other type of medical intervention. It indicated that medical treatment should be used only if it benefited the patient. "There is no duty to continue (life-sustaining machinery) once it has become futile in the opinion of qualified medical personnel" (Paris and Reardon, 1985).

These are only a few of the landmark cases involving passive euthanasia. Each case adds to the guidelines for physicians. Once a landmark decision has been made, however, it does not mean that other decisions always will follow that ruling. Recent medical and legal decisions regarding artificial feeding have created considerable controversy. Situations involving the withholding of nourishment for the terminally ill or the permanently unconscious when their lives are no longer meaningful have placed this issue in the limelight. One result is that some groups are pushing for legislation stipulating that under no circumstances will physicians starve a patient to death (Otten, 1986).

Passive versus Active Euthanasia

People's ideas vary about life, sickness, and death. As a result, numerous reasons are given for allowing or not allowing euthanasia, and if it is not allowed, for the kind of euthanasia practiced: active or passive. Among the reasons for not permitting euthanasia are the following:

- The true condition of a patient may not be known.
- Medicine is rapidly changing and might find a cure for the patient's problems at some future time.
- Families facing financial and emotional burdens may not think rationally about what to do at such times.
- An insurance company may not pay the medical claim if the person ends his or her suffering through euthanasia.
- No policy, law, or legal decision could consider all the variables, and without the proper guidelines, people would be at the mercy of others.

Among the arguments proposing some form of euthanasia are the following:

- The U.S. Constitution gives a person the right to do with his or her body as he or she sees fit.
- A person who is in extreme pain from an incurable illness should not be obliged to prolong suffering to an inevitable death.
- Euthanasia allows organs to be harvested for transplantation before they have been allowed to wither.
- When there is not hope for recovery, prolonging life almost indefinitely can be at the expense of the family or society.

There are people who agree with all the reasons for allowing euthanasia that are cited above. In addition, they state that passive euthanasia is insufficient in some cases. They advocate that active euthanasia should be allowed in some very carefully controlled situations. Arguments for active euthanasia are not articulated very often because the intentional termination of a life is contrary to the medical profession's ethics and against the law.

Nevertheless, some people argue that once the decision is made that a patient has an incurable problem and is suffering extreme pain which cannot be relieved, or is in a vegetative state, active euthanasia is the only humane solution. Regardless of whether treatment is continued or whether the person is allowed to discontinue artificial feeding it may take one to several days before the person dies. Proponents of active euthanasia advocate the use of a lethal injection as a quick, painless, and humane course of action. It would save the person from days of suffering and be more humane for the family as well.

In *Jean's Way*, Derek Humphrey (1978) wrote about his first wife's voluntary euthanasia. He indicated that she spent her last days in a happy manner and chose when she was to die. At the time she chose, he brought her a drink that would end her life. She drank it and apparently was saved from severe discomfort in the last stages of her terminal illness.

In certain countries, physicians have the right to comply with a patient's request for a death medication under very specific circumstances. These countries are Switzerland, Uruguay, Peru, Japan, Germany, and the Netherlands (Koop, 1976 and Humphrey, 1987).

There is another consideration that some people do not like to talk about, **the cost of dying**. Nevertheless, it is an important consideration. About 30 percent of all Medicare costs are contracted in the last year of a person's life. Routine care for someone with a feeding tube is over $13,000 a month. How are people to handle such bills? Is a family to lose all their savings and possessions to keep a person alive in agony? Few people can manage the financial expenditure of maintaining someone in a facility for a long time. Even if they could, there is still the emotional cost of seeing a loved one waste away. Karen Ann Quinlan lived more than nine years without her respirator. She was kept alive by receiving food and water through a feeding tube. When she finally died, she weighed sixty pounds.

The 1985 Harris poll (Mehling, 1986, p. 5) found that 85 percent of the people interviewed believed that terminally ill patients should have their wishes respected regarding how they die. This was a 7 percent increase from 1981 (78 percent) and a 14 percent increase from 1977 (71 percent).

Regardless of the arguments, some people are taking action they feel their conscience compels them to take. These actions are reviewed by the communication media and the courts. Some of the cases are discussed in the following section.

Debbie

An account of a "mercy killing" entitled "It's over, Debbie" was published in the JAMA, a publication of the American Medical Association. A hospital resident described injecting 20 milligrams of morphine into a 20-year-old, terminal cancer patient. The woman was said to have been unable to eat or sleep for over two days because of pain. The resident decided to end her suffering at her request. The resulting controversy involved:

- whether or not the incident ever occurred
- could euthanasia be rationalized
- should the essay have been published.

Bloom, M. (1988). Science. 239:1235-36.

Euthanasia Guidelines in the Netherlands

- The patient must request active euthanasia on his or her own.
- The request must be entirely voluntary.
- The person must have incurable pain.
- A physician who is not connected with the case must review the circumstances and agree that the action should be taken.
- The provision of euthanasia must involve injection.
- The patient's family is unable to make the decision for the patient; this ensures that

Cases Involving Active Euthanasia

This type of euthanasia is practiced considerably less frequent than passive euthanasia, yet some examples do exist. Only a few will be discussed. More than half of the fifty-six mercy killings on record have occurred since 1980.

On June 20, 1973, Lester Zygmaniak shot and killed his brother George who had been paralyzed from the neck down following a motorcycle accident (Heifetz, 1975). George had begged the physicians to let him die. They refused. Then George begged his brother to help him end his suffering. Over a three-day period, he continued to plead with his brother whenever he saw him. Lester had George's wife's support and promise not to interfere. Finally Lester shot his brother. He stood trial and was acquitted, having been found "temporarily insane" owing to sleep deprivation and stress.

The courts are not always so lenient (Trafford and Carey, 1985). A well-known physician named Kreaai gave a man suffering from Alzheimer's disease large injections of insulin. A woman in Virginia used an ice pick to kill her husband who had been suffering from cancer. Both were given jail sentences.

On March 4, 1985, Ros Gilbert fired two bullets into his wife's head. She died immediately. Gilbert said he shot his wife of 51 years out of love and compassion. According to Gilbert, she was in pain from osteoporosis and suffering from Alzheimer's disease. The trial lasted only four days. Gilbert would not say that he was sorry or allow his lawyer to plead temporary insanity. He had taken care of his wife all their married life and felt that he was continuing to do so by putting her out of her misery. The controversy centered around whether or not Gilbert killed his wife for his convenience or because she was suffering from progressively erratic behavior and painful osteoporosis. The jury convicted him of murder, and he was sentenced to 25 years, a life sentence for a 75-year-old man.

Severely Deformed Newborn Children

Another problem associated with euthanasia involves the termination of the life of a severely deformed newborn. As has been discussed, many of the early agricultural and migrating societies were unconcerned about whether a child lived. If a child was deformed in some way, there was little chance that it would be encouraged to live. Martin Luther (1488-1546) and John Calvin (1509-64) deviated from the teaching of Catholicism in their belief that physically and medically deformed infants were made by the devil and had no soul (Althaus, 1972).

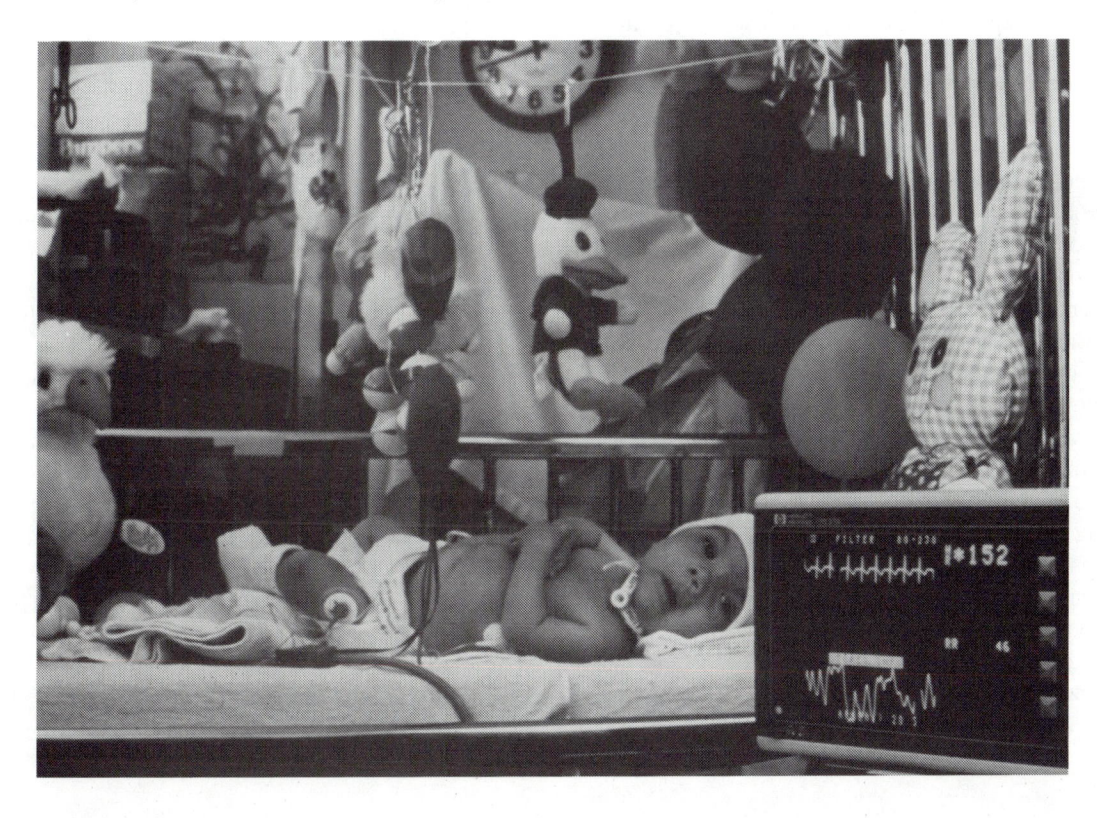

A number of societies practiced infanticide until quite recently. Among the reasons for this practice were that the child had a severe handicap or was of an undesirable gender. Another reason was simply not wanting the child because of inadequate food supply mandated population control.

The thalidomide babies of the 1970s focused the public's attention on severely deformed children. About 8000 malformed babies with shortened or missing limbs were born to women who had taken this presumed safe sedative. Technological advances have enabled physicians to help some deformed children. Nevertheless, intervention is not always used. At Yale University Hospital, 43 of 299 infant deaths appeared to result from a lack of intervention involving the latest technology (Koop, 1976).

Most euthanasia legislation has not applied to anyone under age twenty-one (Rachels, 1975). There was no need. Until recently children with abnormal physical problems died naturally soon after they were born. Even with medical intervention, many children with severe deformities have a hard fight to live.

"Baby Doe" from Bloomington, Indiana, is an example of an infant with an abnormal mental and physical condition (High court, 1986; Neonatologists judge, 1988). This case more than any other has caused legislators to consider that action is needed to protect severely deformed children.

Baby Doe was born April 12, 1982. He had numerous defects including mental retardation, a deformed esophagus, and complications involving the heart. His parents decided against repairing the esophagus and won their case in the lower court. The Supreme Court refused to intervene. Baby Doe died before the petition was reviewed by the U.S. Supreme Court.

Within a month the hospital was threatened with a loss of federal funding if other newborns with similar types of problems were allowed to die without medical treatment or sustenance. Other regulatory notices followed, and legislative efforts currently are under consideration.

In discussing this issue, Tifft (1983) states that pro-life groups lobby to ensure that handicapped children receive every medical consideration for life. Other groups, however, are concerned that regulations could go to extreme lengths and require that all handicapped children be maintained regardless of their condition.

According to Rachels (1975) some physicians refuse to operate on children with Down's syndrome. These physicians cite future misery for those children as their rationale. One explained that many parents want to do everything to keep their child alive yet a few years later institutionalize and ignore the child.

Turbo (1976) states that in Florida approximately 1,500 individuals currently are classified as severely retarded. Many of these children are bedridden. Some are incapable of feeding themselves. The cost of providing care for these children up to age fifty could run from four to six billion dollars.

It might seem easy to make the decision to let a severely deformed child die, to let nature take its course. But this may result in emotional difficulties for many physicians and health care practitioners. According to Shaw (1972), it is extremely difficult to watch a tiny infant wither away with cries that become weaker and weaker. He advocates giving these children a lethal injection to enable them to die without suffering.

International Practices of Euthanasia

Turbo (1976) tells about a severely deformed child who was born in Belgium. His mother, Susan Vandeput, had taken thalidomide during her pregnancy. Once she had the baby at home, the mother put a lethal dose of sedative in the child's bottle. She was charged with infanticide. Her defense was that her child's brain was normal and that he would know what was going on. She felt she could not let her baby suffer through life with such overwhelming deformities. The physician who had given the mother the sedative also stated that he had no remorse. All the defendants were acquitted, and a survey conducted at that time disclosed that 95 percent of the public questioned favored acquitting the mother.

A case in England involved a major in the Royal Corps of Signals (Turbo, 1976). He put his three-month-old Down's syndrome son to death by giving him gas. When this case was tried, the father was found innocent of murder, but he was given a twelve-month imprisonment for manslaughter.

Considerable controversy was generated by Dr. Peter Haemmerli, Chief of Medicine in a Zurich hospital (Culliton, 1975). A number of patients in the department of medicine were alive only in a technical sense, being sustained by nasogastric feeding tubes.

What is generally not known outside the medical profession is that forced feedings can cause comatose patients to gag, retch, and even vomit. Thus, even though patients may be unconscious, forced feedings may not be pleasant for them. Additionally, the tube can cause ulcers and sometimes accompanying bleeding, even hemorrhaging. Dr. Haemmerli and his staff declined to force feed those patients in vegetative states.

A collective decision was made by the support staff on a patient-by-patient basis. The tubes were removed, and the action was charted. The patients were allowed to die comfortably. A visiting physician to the hospital heard about the action and reported it to the authorities. Haemmerli was brought up on charges and cleared. Public sentiment approved.

The Haemmerli case is an example of passive euthanasia. Following is a case of active euthanasia that attracted considerable attention (Weir, 1977). It involved a young physician in Africa. He was caring for his father who was suffering from cancer of the prostate. This disease often metastasizes to the bones and is associated with intense pain. The physician gave his aged father a drug overdose. He said that he did so because he felt that it was the best treatment for him. He had tried morphine and other medications and could not control his father's pain.

At the court trial the son/doctor was found guilty of murder. The judge, however, was in complete sympathy with the actions of the son. He therefore sentenced the man to be detained until he arose from the bench, the "rising of the court." The medical council viewed the case differently and took the doctor's license away for several years.

The Current State of Euthanasia

People hate to let go of their loved ones, and death is often difficult to recognize, especially for a family member. Machines can prolong visible signs of life even after the brain has ceased to function. As summarized by Wanzer et al. (1984, p. 956), "Physicians do not easily accept the concept that it may be best to do less, not more, for a patient. The decision to pull back is much more difficult to make than the decision to push ahead with aggressive support, and today's sophisticated and complex medical technology invites physicians to make use of all the means at their disposal."

Nevertheless, a patient clearly has the right to make decisions about his or her medical treatment. That right is grounded in both common law and the Constitutional right of privacy. When the living will is in place, there should be no problem.

In the case of an incompetent individual, there are desirable steps to consider, according to Oden (1976). First it must be established that the patient would have wished to have no heroic measures taken. Ideally this is evidenced by a living will. The family, guardian, or other immediate next of kin must also be in agreement. Then the attending physician must determine that there is no possibility of the person returning to a cognitive, or thinking, state and resuming a productive life. There might also be irrefutable evidence that death is imminent. All this information is submitted to a hospital ethics committee for its approval.

In a 1988 survey of 5,000 physicians conducted by the Hemlock Society, an advocacy group for euthanasia (Macklin, 1988, p. 4), physicians were screened regarding their attitudes toward euthanasia. Sixty-two percent of the respondents said that "it's sometimes right" for the physician to be involved in assisting terminally ill patients to die. Approximately twenty percent indicated that they had already taken such action.

An ad hoc committee of recognized professionals was established at Harvard (Wanzer et al., 1984) to try to establish guidelines for physicians caring for patients dying of a progressive illness. They designated four levels of care for patients:

1. emergency resuscitation
2. intensive care and advanced life support
3. general medical care, including cancer chemotherapy, artificial hydration, and nutrition
4. general nursing care and efforts to make a patient comfortable, including pain relief, hydration, and nutrition

In the fourth stage, routine monitoring procedures may be discontinued as well as diagnostic measures except when indicated to relieve discomfort. Antibiotics do not have to be given for pneumonia or other infections. Interventions are justified only to make the patient comfortable. Because someone in a terminal condition may not be aware of thirst or hunger, food and water often are of little interest to the patient. The committee agreed that, in the case of a competent patient, sometimes aggressive treatment is advisable, depending on the wishes of the patient. However, for someone in a persistent vegetative state, the above "make the patient comfortable" treatment was judged to be competent medical care. Again, the decision was to be guided by the family or the patient's advocate. Regardless of the treatment, humane kindness was stressed as the bottom line of the health care provided.

Hospitals are now required to establish formal policies regarding resuscitation of terminally ill patients. Nursing homes do not currently have such policies. However, the need is being recognized, and some homes are developing such policies.

Summary

Discussion in this chapter has included information about current and earlier practices of euthanasia in this and other cultures, some religious and legislative considerations, and a review of the number and variety of problems inherent in trying to provide care for a patient with different types of mental and physical problems. Many states and some other countries are all trying to evolve satisfactory ways to work out concerns and problems associated with how a person should die.

Current practices are recognized as temporary and unsatisfactory, and until some universal agreement is reached – which may be a long time from now because of all the different schools of thought associated with euthanasia – this will continue to be a topic involving considerable emotion, from sadness and grief to fear and frustration. An issue as important as this must be recognized as having no simple or easy answer.

One positive note associated with all this chaos, however, is that people care about what is best for the patient. If there were no such concern, there would be no controversy and no evidence of the present chaos about the terminally ill.

Cited References

Althaus, P. (1972). *The Ethics of Martin Luther.* Philadelphia: Fortress Press.

Barnard, C. (1980). *Good life/good death: A doctor's case for euthanasia and suicide.* Englewood Cliffs, N.J.: Prentice-Hall.

Colen, B. D. (1976). *Karen Ann Quinlan. Dying in the age of eternal life.* New York: Nash Publishing.

Culliton, B. J. (1975, December 26). The Haemmerli affair: Is passive euthanasia murder? *Science* 190: 1271-75.

Davis, P. (1984, December). What nurses should do when a patient says, "No, I don't want treatment." *Nursing Life,* 43-44.

Devereux, G. (1955). *Mohave ethnopsychiatry and suicide: the psychiatric disturbance of an Indian tribe.* Bureau of American Ethnology, Bulletin No. 175. Washington, D.C.: Government Printing Office.

Gruman, G. J. (1978). Death and dying: euthanasia and sustaining life. Historical perspective. In *Encyclopedia of Bioethics.* ed. W. T. Reich, pp. 261-68. New York: The Free Press.

Heifetz, M. (1975). *The right to die.* New York: Putnam.

High court says 'no' to administration's Baby Doe rule. (1986, June 27). *Science,* 232: 1595-96.

Humphrey, D., (1987, December 20). Headlines on trial: debate. Topic: Euthanasia. Television program, Today, on ABC.

Humphrey, D., and Wickett, A. (1978). *Jean's Way.* Los Angeles: Hemlock Grove.

Jackson, D. C., and Youngner, S. (1979). Patient autonomy and "death with dignity" – some clinical caveats. *New England Journal of Medicine,* 301: 404-8.

Kennard, E. A. (1937). Hopi reactions to death. *American Anthropologist,* 39: 491-96.

Koop, C. E. (1976). *The right to live: the right to die.* Wheaton, Ill.: Tyndale House of Publishers.

Lo, B. (1984). The death of Clarence Herbert: withdrawing care is not murder. *Annals of Internal Medicine,* 101: 248-51.

Macklin, R. (1988). First Word. *Omni,* 11 (2): 40.

Mehling, A. (1986, July). Developments in living will legislation and significant right to die gains. New York: Society for the Right to Die, 1-5.

Neonatologists judge the Baby Doe regulations. (1988, March 17). *New England Journal of Medicine,* 318: 677-84.

New polls show upward right to die support. (1987, Spring). New York: *Society for the Right to Die,* pp. 1,2.

Oden, T. C. (1976). *Should treatment be terminated? Moral guidelines for Christian families and pastors.* New York: Harper and Row.

Ostheimer, J. M., and Ostheimer, N. C. (1976). *Life and death – who controls?* New York: Springer Publishing.

Otten, A. L. (1986, June 9). Life or death. Issue of force feeding to keep patients alive enters political arena. *The Wall Street Journal.*

Paris, J. J., and Reardon, F. E. (1985, April 19). Court responses to withholding or withdrawing artificial nutrition and fluids. *The Journal of American Medical Association,* 253 (15): 2243-45.

Pius XII, Pope. (1958). The prolongation of life. *The Pope Speaks,* 4: 393-98.

Principles and guidelines concerning the foregoing of life-sustaining treatment of adult patients. (1985). Los Angeles County Medical Association, Committee on Biomedical Ethics. (10 pages.)

Quinlan, J., and Quinlan J., with Beattelle, P. (1977). *Karen Ann.* New York: Doubleday.

Rachels, J. (1975, January 9). Active and passive euthanasia. *The New England Journal of Medicine,* 292 (2): 78-80.

Reynolds, F. E. (1961). Cross-cultural perspectives. W. T. Reich, ed., pp. 229-35. New York: The Free Press.

Right-to-die court decisions. (1988). New York: Society for the Right to Die.

Shaw, A. (1972, January 30). Doctor, do we have a choice? *The New York Times Magazine,* 54.

Simmons, L.W. (1970). *The role of the aged in primitive society.* New York: Archon Books.

Stein, J. J. (1978). *Making medical choices: who is responsible?* Boston: Houghton Mifflin.

Steinbock, B. (1980). *Killing and letting go.* Englewood Cliffs, N.J.: Prentice-Hall.

Tifft, S. (1983, April 11). Debate on the boundary of life. *Time,* 68-70.

Trafford, A., and Carey, J. (1985, September 9). Mercy killings: where theory and reality clash. *U. S. News and World Report,* 27.

Turbo, R. (1976). *An act of mercy: euthanasia today.* Los Angeles: Nash Publishing.

Veatch, R. M. (1978). Professional and public policies. In *Encyclopedia of Bioethics,* W. T. Reich, ed., pp. 278-86. New York: Free Press.

Wanzer, S. H.; Adelstine, S. J.; Cranford, R. D.; Federman, D. D.; Hook, E. D.; Moertel, C. G.; Safar, R.; Stone, A.; Taussig, H. B.; and van Eys, J. (1984). The physician's responsibility toward hopelessly ill patients. *The New England Journal of Medicine,* 310: 955-59.

Warner, W. L. (1937). *A black civilization: a study of an Australian Tribe.* New York: Harper Brothers.

Weir, R. (1977). *Ethical issues in death and dying.* New York: Columbia University Press.

CEO with Cancer

A young man in the prime of life develops cancer of the prostate. He has a very stressful position as the CEO of a large metropolitan store. He is married to a very attractive woman, and they have two children. His mother lives in the same community.

Following the operation to confirm the diagnosis of cancer, the physician recommends to the wife that her husband receive chemotherapy. His wife declines. She also states that she does not want her husband to know that he has cancer.

The conversation is overheard by the patient's mother, who becomes very upset. The mother contacts the doctor and says that the reason the wife does not want the diagnosis disclosed and any treatment is that the wife has a lover.

- Should the doctor tell the wife what her mother-in-law has said and try to determine if the statement is true?

- Does the doctor have a responsibility to tell the diagnosis to the patient and ask him if he wants to have chemotherapy?

- Should a patient have the right to refuse to have chemotherapy?

- If the doctor does follow the wife's wishes, should the mother tell her son?

- With respect to the diagnosis, what advice should the mother give her son if no children were involved?

- Should the mother tell her son about his wife's lover no matter what?

- Should the mother tell her son about the diagnosis and urge him to receive treatment?

- What should the children be told about their father's condition?

- If the doctor were a friend of the husband or the wife, would this have any impact on the decision to tell the patient?

- In order to protect her son's interests and her grandchildren, how can the mother go about gaining power of attorney without telling her son about his wife's lover?

- Does a mother have a right to interfere in the marriage of her son and his wife?

- Should there be a law that states a patient must be told of his/her condition and informed of possible treatment?

- Should the mother take the wife to court after her son dies to get custody of the children based on the restriction the wife placed on the doctor regarding her husband's care?

- What legal recourse does the wife have to control her mother-in-law's interference regarding telling the son/husband about his diagnosis and care?

- Suppose the patient asks the nursing staff about his diagnosis. How should they respond?

- Suppose the doctor does as the wife asks, can the mother request another doctor to intervene?

- Suppose the patient's spiritual leader comes to visit and the patient asks about his diagnosis, what should the clergyman or woman do?

11

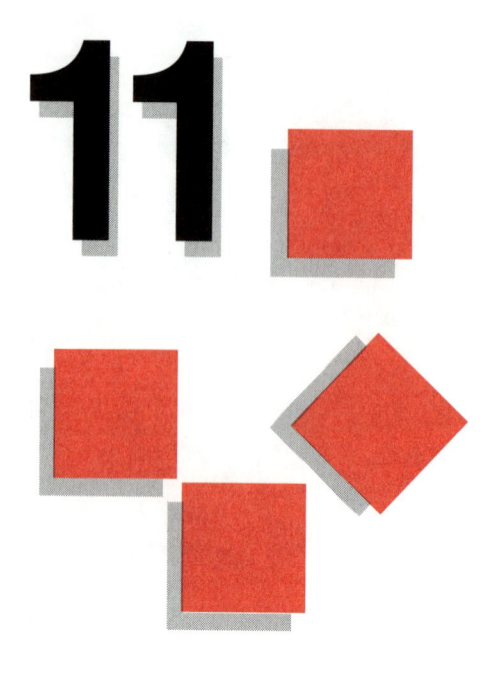

Infanticide: An Ethical Dilemma

Norma J. Walters*

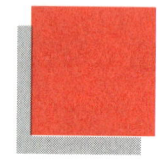

Objectives

After reading this chapter, you should be able to:

- Define the terms listed at the beginning of this chapter.
- Name the act that outlaws discrimination on the basis of handicap.
- List the provisions of the Child Abuse Amendment.
- State the purpose of the Criminal Attempts Act.
- Explain the provisions of the Supreme Court decision that was responsible for legalizing abortion.
- List five reasons for infanticide as revealed by ethicists.
- Explain infanticide-on-demand.
- Describe the two types of cases that advocate euthanasia.
- State the purpose of an ethics committee.
- Review case reports and explain the ethical dilemmas.

Terms and Definitions

- **Active euthanasia.** Hastening death.
- **Infanticide.** Killing of an infant.
- **Neonaticide.** Parents killing an infant.

Introduction

This chapter presents an overview of general information relating to infanticide. Discussion is centered on:
- past and present infanticide
- legislation and infanticide
- ethical decision making and dilemmas
- treatment or nontreatment of handicapped infants
- abortion or the unwanted child
- infant euthanasia
- weighing the cost
- maternity care and cost
- neonatal intensive care
- cost-benefit analysis for low birth-weight infants
- ethics committees.

In addition, several case reports with pros and cons and dilemmas are provided for discussion.

The killing/letting die controversy must qualify as one of the stickier problems in ethics, and the impact on the health professions creates an ethical dilemma in practice. Doctors, nurses, and other health care professionals are constantly grappling with these medical treatment decisions.

---

*Norma J. Walters
Associate Professor and Coordinator, Health Occupations Education, Auburn University, Auburn, AL 36830.

Past and Present Infanticide

Infanticide, as defined by Taber's Cyclopedic Medical Dictionary (1985), is "the killing of an infant, or one who takes the life of an infant." Manney and Blattner (1985) reported that some parents and their agents have been involved in infanticide for centuries. In the past, many parents have taken care of this gruesome ordeal themselves. Peoples living on the edges of survival, such as the Eskimos, have often disposed of babies with physical defects by exposing them to the elements. In other cultures, such as the Chinese, a strong bias in favor of male children has often led to the killing of unwanted female babies.

The authors further revealed that current-day infanticide in the United States usually happens in the hospital. Occasionally, handicapped infants are killed by a direct act, but more often by withholding something the babies need in order to survive. Sometimes a surgical procedure is not performed on a baby even though it is needed for survival (such an operation would always be performed on a "normal" baby). Sometimes water and food are withheld; sometimes large doses of drugs are used to sedate babies so that they will quietly starve without crying in hunger for food. In addition, infections may not be treated by withholding antibiotics, or the life-support system may be discontinued because someone made the decision that the infant was "struggling" and the "quality of life" would not be adequate.

Legislation and Infanticide

The offense of infanticide was first introduced into the Law of England and Wales in 1922 and further amended in 1938. Parker and Good (1981) reported the Infanticide Act ameliorated the judicial process with regard to women who kill their babies. The 1938 Act states that in cases where the woman has a mental imbalance attributable to the birth, the charge is reduced to manslaughter, rather than murder, and the punishment is reduced accordingly.

"Where a woman by any willful act or omission causes the death of her child under the age of twelve months, but at the time of the act or omission the balance of her mind was disturbed by reason of her not having fully recovered from the effect of giving birth to the child or by reason of the effect of lactation consequent upon the birth of the child, then not withstanding that the circumstances were such that the offense would have amounted to murder, she shall be guilty . . . of infanticide and may . . . be dealt with and punished as if she had been guilty of the offense of manslaughter of the child." (p. 239).

The Infanticide Act is unique in two respects:

- It applies only to women.

- It provides a special defense for what was a capital offense, murder, in which the question of responsibility is bypassed.

It must be shown that a mother suffered from a mental imbalance attributable to the effect of giving birth or the consequent action for a verdict of infanticide to be returned. This verdict places the sentencing at the discretion of the judge. However, provisions for attempted infanticide were omitted until a plea of guilty to attempting infanticide under the Criminal Attempts Act of 1981 was accepted by the court.

In 1983, the United States Department of Health and Human Services (HHS) began to operate a twenty-four-hour toll-free "hotline" set up by the regulations for reporting – anonymously – any case in which a handicapped newborn infant is denied care or nutrition (the Baby Doe regulations). However, the court struck down the regulation.

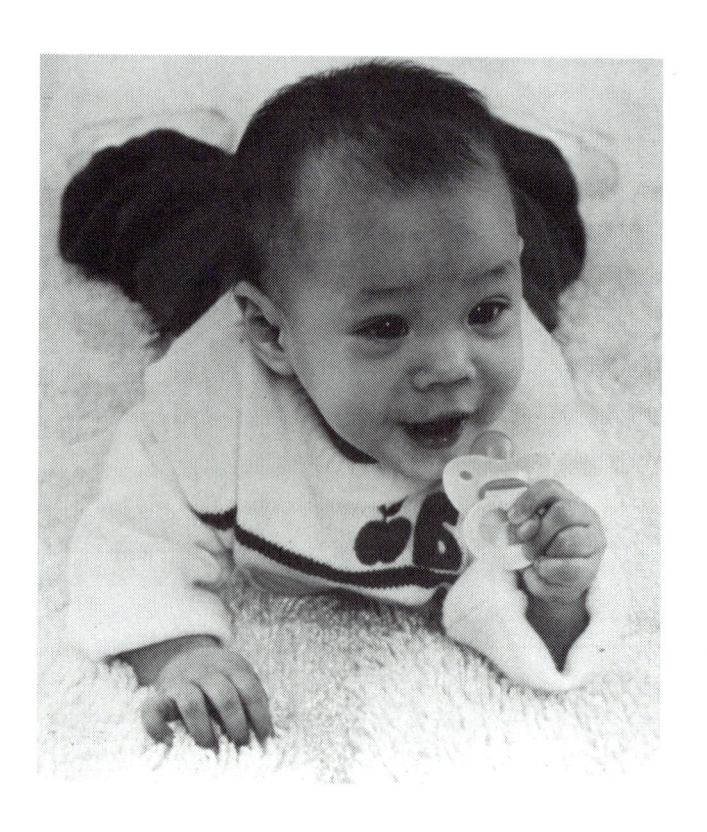

Rehabilitation Act

According to Section 504 of the Rehabilitation Act of 1973, which outlaws discrimination on the basis of handicap, hospitals were required to post notice of a hotline in all newborn nurseries and neonatal intensive care units (ICUs). "Hospitals that failed to follow through, or that denied the requisite care, could lose Medicare and Medicaid funds" (News: HHS, 1983. p. 851). The United States Department of Heath, Education, and Welfare (HEW), the predecessor of HHS, had adopted the position that 504 did not give it authority to regulate actions regarding patients' rights "to receive or refuse treatment."

Rather, HEW's authority was to make services "accessible" or available to the handicapped, so as to provide them with "an equal opportunity to receive benefits" (Annas, 1984. p. 728); HEW explained the difference:

"A burn center need not provide other types of medical treatment to handicapped persons unless it provides such medical services to non-handicapped persons. It could not, however, refuse to treat the burns of a deaf person because of his or her deafness."

"In fact, it was not until the May 1982 letter to hospitals that HHS ever suggested that 504 might reach to actual medical treatment decisions" (Annas, 1984, p. 618). After reviewing the Baby Doe regulations, the court found that "the regulatory history of 504 was inconclusive," of the enabling statute and was "flatly at odds with the position originally taken by HEW" (p. 728). This left the court to interpret the statute based on its language and legislative history. Cited in Annas (1984), Section 504 stated:

"No otherwise qualified handicapped individual in the United States . . . shall, solely by reason of his handicap, be excluded from the participation in or be denied the benefits of, or be subjected to discrimination under any program or activity receiving Federal financial assistance."

The court concluded, therefore, "that the Rehabilitation Act did not give HHS any authority to interfere with treatment decisions involving defective newborn infants" (Annas, 1984, p. 728). A big question remained, "What should the role of the government be in treatment decisions for handicapped newborns?" Incidentally, about this time, the Child Abuse Amendment provided assistance.

Hydrocephalic/Down's Syndrome Child

A hydrocephalic Down's syndrome child is always news in a hospital. When the chief-of-staff's sister had such a baby, everyone knew about it. The baby was full-term, approximately nine pounds, and grossly deformed.

Immediately following the delivery and a conference with the parents, the chief-of-staff indicated that the baby was not to be fed anything and preparations were made for the baby to be discharged.

What is the reasoning behind these actions, and what responsibility, if any, should you have if you were a member of the health care team at that hospital?

Child Abuse Amendment

HR 1904, the Child Abuse Amendment of 1984, provided that state child protective service agencies, health care facilities, and health professionals develop procedures to ensure that medically indicated treatment, nutrition (including fluid maintenance), general care, and social services as appropriate, be provided to infants at risk with life-threatening congenital impairments. The Act also included specific requirements for HHS to:

- publish guidelines to encourage and assist health care providers desiring to establish local health care mechanisms for the review of care provided to infants at risk with life-threatening congenital impairments

- develop a directory of available medical and community resources

- determine the most effective means of supporting the medical treatment of such infants financially.

This direction empowered the federal government only to support state abuse efforts with financial and technical information and not to become directly involved in individual cases (Annas, 1984).

Fetal Abuse

The 1973 Supreme Court decision Roe vs. Wade did more than legalize abortion. It stipulated an implied two-pronged obligation on the part of a woman. If a woman chose not to have an abortion, she would be obligated to provide the best possible environment for her child, in and out of the womb. If, on the other hand, a woman refused to discontinue activities or habits proven dangerous to a fetus, it would be her obligation to abort the unborn child (Benson, 1984).

State and Federal Medicaid for Abortion

Before the Supreme Court legalized abortion throughout the country in 1973, only a handful of state Medicaid programs covered abortion, unless the procedure was necessary to save the woman's life (Robinson et al., 1974). However, there were no restrictions on the federal Medicaid payments for abortion until 1976, when Congress passed the Hyde Amendment, limiting reimbursements to abortions needed to save the woman's life. Except for the first seven months of 1980 (when Medicaid funding resumed), federal payments for abortion have been severely restricted. The Hyde Amendment added new versions in 1976 and 1979 to permit funding when a pregnancy resulted from rape or incest, if the crime was promptly reported to law enforcement officials, or if two physicians confirmed that the woman would suffer severe and long-lasting physical health damage if her pregnancy was continued. The physical health damage criterion was dropped in 1980. Since June 1981, abortions have been reimbursable under Medicaid only if the woman's life would be endangered by carrying the pregnancy to term.

Despite legislation, ethics committees, thoughts of health care professionals, right-to-life groups, or other individuals, the concern continues and the question regarding infanticide may not always be answered to everyone's satisfaction. Whether it is **neonaticide** (parents killing an infant) or **active euthanasia** (hastening the infant's death), the question remains, "Is infanticide right or wrong?"

Ethical Decision Making and Dilemmas

Ethical thinking of the medical profession regarding the quality of life is being dominated by a new scheme of ethics. This "new medical ethic" was described in *California Medicine* in 1970. The anonymous editorialist thought that the medical profession was caught between two ethics:

- The old ethic, nurtured by the Judeo-Christian moral tradition, placed great emphasis on the intrinsic worth and equal value of every human life regardless of its stage or condition.

- New quality-of-life ethic would make it necessary and acceptable to place relative rather than absolute values on such things as human lives.

In the past, babies have been killed for all the reasons cited by the anonymous author:

- because others think a handicapped infant's life is not worth living.

- because the burdens of raising handicapped children will interfere with the personal well-being of their parents and siblings.

- because disabled people are unproductive and expensive social burdens.

Infanticide on Demand

The theologian Joseph Fletcher (1972) is often quoted by physicians who advocate infanticide on demand. Fletcher believes that infanticide is acceptable because human beings have a moral obligation to increase human well-being wherever possible and that "all rights are imperfect and can be set aside if human need requires it."

Suicide and mercy killing are acceptable in this scheme, as is infanticide. Such acts are not regrettable necessities or grim compromises with one's conscience, but positive human goods (cited in Manney and Blattner, 1985). Fletcher also writes "that in some situations a morally good end can justify a relatively bad means" (1980).

Treatment or Nontreatment of Handicapped Infants

Ethicists relate other reasons for infanticide. Some simply think that impaired babies are not human persons. One philosopher, Michael Tooley (1972) of Stanford University, reported that it is unfortunate that

---

Quality of Life Formula

One study on babies with spina bifida reported the following: A team of doctors and other clinicians, using a quality of life formula, recommended that 24 of 69 babies born with spina bifida between 1977 and 1982 not be aggressively treated. The 24 untreated babies died at an average of 37 days. Of those who were recommended for aggressive treatment, all lived except one killed in a car accident. Of those not recommended for treatment, six of eight babies whose parents went ahead with treatment lived. The treatment recommendations were based in part on the child's expected "quality of life." (QL). This was formulated by multiplying the child's natural environment (NE) with the sum of the financial and emotional contribution expected from the child's home (H) and society (S).

$$QL = NE \times (H + S)$$

The results of this study have caused considerable controversy.

Creighton, 1984, pp. 16-17.

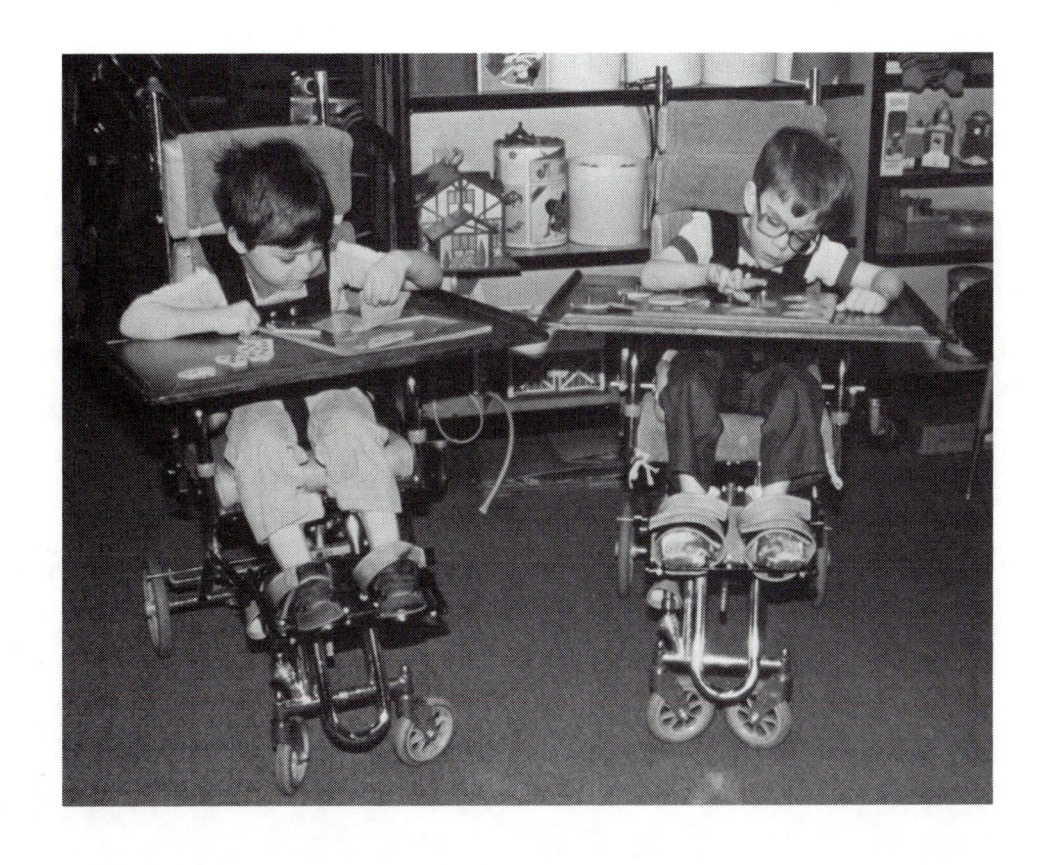

most people use the terms **person** and **human being** interchangeably. Tooley says persons have rights (including the right to life); however, not every human being can properly be regarded as a person. His rule: "An organism possesses the concept of experiences and other mental states, and believes that it is itself such a continuing entity" (p. 37). With this philosophy, Tooley would allow infanticide up to a week after birth.

If Tooley doubts the personhood of the handicapped baby, Joseph Fletcher (1972) doubts even the child's humanity. Fletcher has confused the modernist with about fifteen criteria to make the critical judgment whether someone is human. Some of these include:

- a minimal intelligence
- a sense of future
- a sense of the past
- a capacity to relate to others
- a balance between rationality and feeling.

Fletcher is very specific about some criteria and very vague about others. For example, a human being with an IQ of 40 is considered only questionably a person, and if the IQ is below 20, he or she is definitely not a person.

Other ethicists more subtle than Tooley and Fletcher have exercised great influence on medical thinking about these questions, and many of their answers have been equally unsatisfactory. A common reaction to opinions by Tooley and Fletcher would be to dismiss them as grotesque musings by eccentric academics. However, they are an important part of the puzzle of infanticide and its growing acceptance.

Specialists in Bioethics

Doctors look to specialists in bioethics for guidance in their treatment of newborns who are handicapped. So do policymakers, parents, and hospital administrators. In the past, theologians and philosophers have been involved with the federal government commission that sanctioned experimentation on unborn babies scheduled for abortion, and on the presidential commission in 1983 that decided that stiffer penalties were not necessary to stop infanticide.

Relational Principle for Handicapped Newborns

Years ago, McCormick (1974), writing in the *Journal of the American Medical Association* gave a relational principle for the handicapped newborns. A life that is "painful, poverty-stricken and deprived, away from home and friends, oppressive, may be a life of which it could be said that human relationships – which are the very possibility of growth in love of God and neighbor – would be so threatened, strained or submerged that they would no longer function as the heart meaning of the individual's life as they should" (p. 173). The Christian can say, in these cases, that life has achieved its potential and the individual can be allowed to die.

McCormick hoped that these guidelines would assist in making decisions about sustaining the lives of grossly deformed and deprived infants. However, his guidelines raised many questions, such as:

- How can healthy adults with no experience of disabilities imagine the quality and value of relationships a handicapped baby might have in future years?

- What do **grossly deformed** and **deprived** mean?

The relationship principle does not compel anyone to agree with McCormick. However, Horan (1980) reports that "there is no way that the relational principle can be less than a death warrant for some retardates except in the hands of McCormick himself" (p. 198). The principle falls apart as someone begins to apply it to specific cases. However, in 1983 McCormick co-authored with Paris, "Saving Defective Infants: Options for Life or Death" and presented more cautions since infanticide had become more common. These included:

- Babies should not die because their families cannot cope with them.

- Retarded babies should not be left to starve because they are retarded.

- Nontreatment decisions are not private matters as doctors claim.

- The courts can properly intervene when decision makers behave irresponsibly.

Life-and-Death Decisions

Life-and-death decisions create an ethical dilemma for doctors, nurses, parents, and other health care professionals. "To treat or not to treat" infants is a judgment made by someone. Despite the benefits that respirators and other lifesaving equipment provide, doctors don't know if aggressive health care will help infants get better or merely extend their existence. Infants with an unclear prognosis can put parents and health professionals in a tough position. Physicians don't want to prolong the suffering of an incurably ill newborn, yet they are dedicated to helping babies survive (Fackelmann, 1986).

In addition to the handicapped infant, there is the issue of abortion or the unwanted child, which has raised the question of rights and moral behaviors. These issues have been in controversy for several years.

Abortion or the Unwanted Child

Dr. James Prescott (1976), from the National Institute of Child Health and Human Development, pointed out that the questions of abortion and moral behavior are unlikely to be resolved by religious convictions, or theological doctrine, since such convictions and doctrine vary considerably among free people and are, at best, arbitrary in their formation and implementation. The antiabortion movement believes that, even in the embryonic stage of development, the fetus is a human life and that any deliberate termination of embryonic or fetal life is unjustified – that is, homicide. Conversely, proponents of abortion deny, particularly during the embryonic stage of development, that a fetus is a human life. Therefore they believe that the termination of fetal life does not constitute homicide.

In addition, proponents of abortion justify termination of a fetal life by asserting:

- that the woman has the ultimate right to control her own body

- that no individual or group of individuals has any right to force a woman to carry a pregnancy that she does not want

- that parents have the moral responsibility and constitutional obligation to bring into this world only children who are wanted and loved

- that children have certain basic human and constitutional rights, for example, the right to have loving, caring parents, sound health, and protection from harm.

Conflicts of Rights of Fetus

Prescott also reported that conflicts of rights of the fetus, the rights of the woman, the rights of the child, the rights of adults to unlimited reproduction, and the rights of society need very careful consideration in evaluating the morality of abortion. These rights bring many questions which have been unanswered. As reported, these may include:

- Do adults who are incapable of responsible behavior (mentally retarded, for example) have the right to become pregnant and bring children into this world who most probably would be neglected and/or abused and who will possibly become infant- and child-mortality statistics?

- Do mentally retarded individuals have the right to parentage?

Consequences of Denied Abortions

In one report, the development of children from birth to age twenty-one was examined. The sample included 121 children who were compared with a control group of children whose mothers had not applied for abortion. In the unwanted group, 17 percent were born out of wedlock, versus only 7 percent of the control group. The statistically significant differences are summarized as follows:

- 60 percent of children who were classified as unwanted had an insecure childhood versus 28 percent of the control group. (Insecure childhood would be unsatisfactory home conditions, moving from home to home, parents divorced or deceased by the time the child was age 15, and born out of wedlock and never legitimized.)

- 28 percent of children classified as unwanted had received some form of psychiatric care, compared with 15 percent of the control group.

- 18 percent of children classified as unwanted were registered with child-welfare boards for some type of delinquency, whereas, only 8 percent of the control group.

- 14 percent of children classified as unwanted received some type of welfare during the ages of 16 and 21, versus 2.5 percent of the control group.

- 14 percent of children classified as unwanted had some type of higher education, compared to 33 percent of the control group.

- 68 percent of the control group children did not show any of the social disabilities mentioned above, versus only 48 percent of the children classified as unwanted.

In brief, children who were classified as unwanted were found to be more than twice as likely to suffer emotional, social, and educational disadvantages as children classified as wanted. In addition, children classified as unwanted appeared to present certain costs to their society such as an increased delinquency rate, a higher number of them were welfare cases, a higher number were poorly educated, and a greater percentage had psychiatric problems. According to the researchers, these results strongly support the right of the woman to be pregnant by choice and to be a mother by choice as essential prerequisites for a humane and compassionate society.

Prescott, 1976, pp. 62-67

- Is it not more moral and humane to prevent a life rather than permit a life which may experience suffering and/or deprivation and possibly a brutal early death, which is reflected in child abuse and infant- and child-mortality statistics?
- Is mere physical existence society's highest goal and greatest moral burden or is the quality of human life society's highest goal and greatest moral burden?
- What are the moral and social criteria which should be identified to justify the sacrifice of human life?

Female versus Male Infanticide

A number of cultures have practiced the killing of female infants because they are valued less than male infants. In addition, it has been reported that the People's Republic of China may have an apparent growth in female infanticide and possibly the use of amniocentesis for the determination of sex. This may be one result of the pressure for the one-child campaign. One clinic reported that amniocentesis and antenatal sex determination had come to their rescue and could help in keeping some check over the accelerating population as well as give relief to the couple requiring a male child (Jeffrey et al., 1984). These patterns could have a direct link between more female infanticide and female neglect leading to higher infant and child mortality rates and more frequent termination of pregnancies involving a female fetus.

Infant Euthanasia

The killing/letting die controversy must qualify as one of the most difficult problems in bioethics (Murray, 1985, p. 1106). There are two types of cases where some are inclined to advocate infant euthanasia:

1. The first type is evidence that the infant will die relatively soon anyway, no matter what is done. However, this death can be prolonged if certain treatment is initiated. This treatment may be extraordinary, such as the use of a respirator or the performance of routine surgery. In either case, if nothing is done, the child will die immediately; or if the treatment is initiated, it is believed that the child will live longer but will die in a relatively short time.

2. In the second type, the infant can be saved but at great expense. If nothing is done, the infant will probably die soon. However, if treatment is initiated, the infant will be able to live more or less indefinitely. The expense incurred is the great burden that must be born if the infant is saved. Financial and emotional burdens will fall on the parents and may also burden the infant.

Weir (cited in Murray, 1985) reported that there are three necessary and jointly sufficient conditions for active infant euthanasia:

- that it be responsibly determined that life-prolonging treatment is not in the best interests of the child
- that the child would otherwise endure prolonged suffering
- that the killing be carried out quickly and painlessly.

There are circumstances where society does agree with the taking of life, such as in war or in defense, possibly against an unprovoked and life-threatening attacker. Even in war, we distinguish among those who can be killed – combatants – and those who cannot – noncombatants, including civilians and prisoners of war. However, some may not agree with Weir's conclusion, probably because his conception of the issue is too narrow.

Weighing the Cost

Doctors, nurses, and other health care professionals are constantly grappling with medical treatment decisions every day. They are pressured by a variety of factors, including the catastrophic costs of care. Health care costs now consume in excess of 10 percent of the gross national product. Physicians must balance the benefits of using a procedure with the expense in today's hospitals. Certain patients may never receive potentially lifesaving care because they are judged to be unlikely to recover. There are others who may not receive expensive treatments because their families do not have insurance or money.

Physicians say treatment decisions are going to be even more difficult as technical breakthroughs allow them to save very tiny babies. Even though the public's attention has been focused on the multiple handicapped Down's syndrome babies, low birth-weight infants pose the greater problem for health professionals. Surgery, physicians say, can be predicted; however, tiny newborns often have multiple problems, and it's difficult to identify the infants who will prosper after they are given the appropriate medical care, as reported by Arthur Kohrman, M. D., chairman of the pediatric ethics committee at the University of Chicago.

Health professionals say they are under increasing pressure to stop care when babies are irreversibly ill. Newborns with low birth weight can have hospital bills of $1,000 a day in an intensive care unit, with only a portion paid by Medicaid because federal and state health programs do not pay the entire amount. The result is uncompensated care for a hospital. Some financially squeezed hospitals may be forced to draft no-treatment-guidelines for hopelessly ill newborns as they become less able to absorb the unpaid medical bills. Is it possible that some may decide to end care without parental consent when babies can no longer be helped?

Maternity Care: Patients and Cost

Researchers at the National Bureau of Economic Research reported that Medicaid-subsidized deliveries each year involve nearly 542,000 low-income women. Federal and state governments together have spent billions of dollars throughout the year for Medicaid maternity care. The largest component of maternity care payments is hospitalization (Kenny et al., 1986).

Neonatal Intensive Care

The National Institute of Medicine (1985) revealed that Medicaid payments for neonatal intensive care expenditures vary from state to state throughout the nation. The authors concluded that reducing the need for neonatal intensive care would dramatically lower Medicaid expenditures for the first year of life. Increased use of prenatal care could also be expected to reduce demand for neonatal intensive care by improving pregnancy outcome.

However, according to Brown (1989), participation in prenatal care services in the United States is low relative to that in many other developed countries, and rates of use are declining among some high risk groups. Brown continues, "The major barriers to obtaining prenatal care are inadequate insurance coverage, limitations in the Medicaid program, inadequate capacity in the maternity care system, lack of coordination between health and social services for low-income women, and inhospitable conditions at some sites where prenatal care is delivered."

Cost-Benefit Analysis for Low Birth-Weight Infants

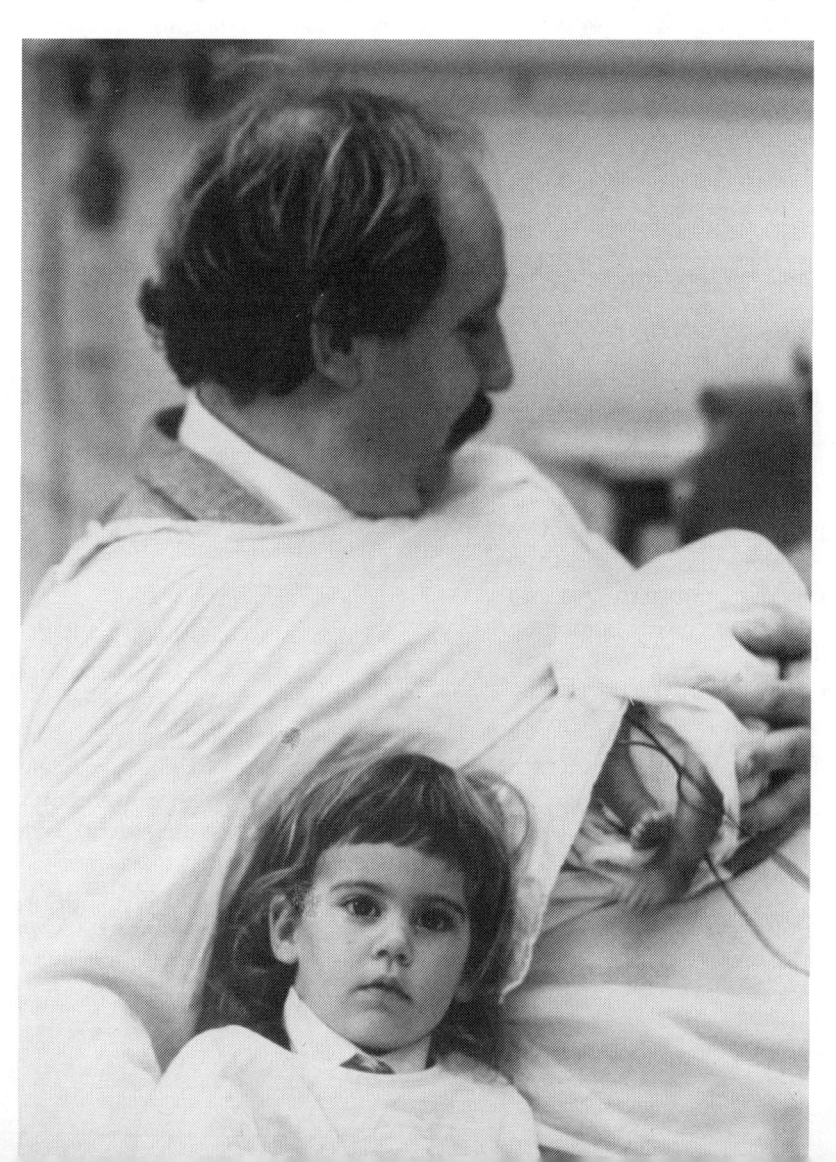

In a study cited in "Death by Design of Handicapped Newborns: The Family's Role and Response" (Rue, 1985), an attempt was made to simplify and reduce decision making regarding "at risk" infants to a cost-benefit analysis, which presumably can be applied to any infant decision-making treatment. Based upon birth weight and economic benefit, infants of 900 grams (g) or greater are approvingly selected for life. Data are shown in the accompanying table.

Death by Design of Infants at Risk for Economic Benefit:

Cost-Benefit Analysis for Low Birth-Weight Infants

Birth Weight (g)	Total Cost/ Survivor*	Average Lifetime Earnings	Expense Income Differential	Optimum Decision Outcome
500-599	---	0	0	DEATH
600-699	$362,992	0	0	DEATH
700-799	$116,221	$55,138	-$61,083	DEATH
800-899	$101,356	$49,887	-51,469	DEATH
900-999	$ 40,647	$77,031	+36,384	LIFE

*Sum of projected hospital, physician, long-term care costs.

NOTE: *This table was made to simplify and reduce decision making regarding "at risk" infants to a cost-benefit analysis, which presumably can be applied to any infant decision-making treatment. Based upon birth and economic benefit, infants of 900 grams or greater are approvingly selected for life. The decision is clear: death by design (Rue, 1985).*

Curiously, 32 percent of infants weighing 500-1,000 g survived, with 72 percent being normal or minimally handicapped in this study. From low birth-weight infants to those born with mental retardation, cerebral palsy, spina bifida, blindness, and loss of limb, the decision is brutally clear: death by design for economic benefit. The author noted that it is possible that the elimination of other types of "dependents" might also be considered such as: unemployed students, grandparents, and uneducated minorities, because of the heavy burden on families and their increasing demands on our municipal services and increasing taxes as well. Margaret Sanger (cited in Rue), founder of Planned Parenthood, prophesied years ago in *The Pivot of Civilization* (1922):

> *". . . the most urgent problem today is how to limit and discourage the over fertility of the mentally and physically defective. Possibly drastic and Spartan measures may be forced upon American society."*

Ethics Committees/Panels

Many hospitals have been spurred to form ethics panels or committees owing to an increasingly complex medical world. These groups of doctors, nurses, lawyers, and members of the community advise parents who are struggling to make a decision. Some evidence suggests that hospital administrators are forming ethics panels or committees before a problem case arises. A 1985 survey by the American Academy of Pediatrics of hospitals with neonatal care units found that nearly 66 percent had an ethics committee (Fackelmann, 1986).

The extensive debates in today's society clearly indicate that no religious, philosophical, or scientific consensus exists concerning the question of whether fetal life is human life, or which handicapped infant should survive. These situations create many dilemmas for health care professionals.

Many times the decisions are just too tough to be handled without guidance provided by medical ethics experts. During early 1986, physicians at Presbyterian-University Hospital in Pittsburgh, Pennsylvania wrote an article in *Critical Care Medicine* that urged hospitals to adopt policies to help doctors and nurses who must work with seriously ill newborns or adults. The authors reported that health care workers can be placed in a legal limbo, even though 80 percent of state legislatures have passed a natural death act. The guidelines the physicians designed and included in their report were intended to assist physicians in making these tough judgment calls.

Case Reports, Pros-Cons, and Dilemmas

Certain cases in the literature relating to treatment versus nontreatment of infants provide examples of ethical dilemmas. Some of these are described below:

Case 1

The original "Baby Doe" case occurred in 1982. A baby born with Down's syndrome and other anomalies required surgery. The parents chose not to permit surgery and requested that the infant not be provided nourishment or any life-support treatment; the infant was allowed to die at the parent's request. This case has prompted an attempt to secure assurance that lives of handicapped children would be protected even against wishes of family. Guidelines were provided to all the hospitals (5,800) that receive federal funding.

Even though the parents refused the surgery and the hospital asked the court for guidance and the baby died six days after the appeal, Carolyn Murphy says the American Nurses Association (ANA) Ethics Committee "would agree that it's a dangerous thing to make rash decisions about the quality of life possible for some handicapped infants." "On the other hand, some of these children are born with multiple anomalies and keeping them alive may mean subjecting them to prolonged suffering" (News: HHS stands by, 1983, p. 869).

Case 2

Baby Jane Doe, born in 1983, the first child of young parents who were married one year, suffered from spina bifida, hydrocephaly, and microcephaly. Physicians recommended immediate surgery to reduce the fluid in her skull and close the meningomyelocele. With this procedure performed, life expectancy could possibly be increased from a few weeks to twenty years. However, she would likely be severely retarded, bedridden, paralyzed, epileptic, and subject to constant urinary tract infections. The parents refused to consent to surgery after lengthy consultations, opting for antibiotics and bandages for prevention of infection. The physicians disagreed.

A Vermont right-to-life lawyer filed suit to obtain an order for surgery to be performed, and the trial judge appointed an attorney to represent the child. The attorney agreed with the parents and then reversed his decision at the hearing because medical records disagreed with the prognosis given by physicians to the parents. The trial judge ruled the infant was in need of immediate surgery. However, the parents appealed. The Appellate Division reversed the decision of the judge, "ruling that the parents' decision was consistent with the best interests of the child" (Annas, p. 727). Later, the New York Court of Appeals ruled that allegations of child abuse or neglect must be made to the state's Department of Social Services; and dismissed the suit.

The United States Department of Health and Human Services (HHS) received a hotline complaint about this time and referred it to the New York Child Protection Services. The Child Protection Service concluded that there was no cause for state intervention. Surgeon General C. Everett Koop concluded after reviewing the records, that he could not determine the basis for denial of treatment. Under Section 504, HHS brought suit in U. S. District Court to get the child's records. The District Court concluded that the hospital failed to perform the surgery not because of the child's handicap, but because of parental refusal; therefore, the hospital was not in violation (Annas, p. 727). HHS appealed; the Court of Appeals concluded that Baby Jane Doe fit the definition of a "handicapped individual," but determined she was not "otherwise qualified," because this phrase referred to handicapped individuals who could benefit from the services in spite of their handicap rather than cases in which the handicap itself is the subject of service (Annas, 1984, p. 728).

Case 3

Siamese twins, joined at the waist and sharing the lower stomach and bowels were gasping for air at birth. The anesthesiologist said, "Ventilate;" the other doctor, who was called to assist with the difficult birth, said, "Don't resuscitate, let's cover the babies." A nurse turned off the oxygen and went to the nurses lounge where she "sat down in shock," as reported in the *New York Times,* July 2, 1981. The twins survived the birth, and the doctor allegedly gave orders not to feed them in accordance with a request from the parents. Witnesses could not link the parents with any orders to withhold food or medical care; however, a medical chart was presented by the state with the entry "Do not feed infants, in accordance with parents' wishes." The judge ruled that as hearsay and excluded it from testimony. At

---

Infant Deaths

Of 299 deaths over a 2.5-year period, forty-three (14 percent) deaths in the special-care nursery occurred "after parents and physicians jointly agreed to discontinue treatment because of multiple anomalies, meningomyelocele, cardiopulmonary crippling, or other central nervous system defects. The remaining 256 who received the best treatment modern medicine and nursing could provide lived little, if any longer, than those who received no special treatment. For each of the forty-three babies for whom no further treatment was given, the physicians and parents made a decision that the prognosis was very poor or hopeless for meaningful life. The awesome finality of these decisions, combined with a potential for error in prognosis, made the choice agonizing for families and health professionals"

Creighton, 1984, p. 16

the custody hearing, the judge upheld the state's contention that the twins had been indeed denied food, water, and medical care. However, he did not rule on "who was responsible for the abuse" (Horan, 1982, p. 75). That was the central issue remaining in the criminal charge against the parents and physician.

The state was awarded custody of the twins, and the judge said that the right to live is given even to newborn Siamese twins with severe anomalies. He also asked: "Has society retrogressed to the stage where we mortals can say to a newborn abnormal child, you have no right to live with a little help from us? I hope not and think not, although the evidence in this case goes on to contradict me" (Horan, 1982, p. 75).

In Horan's article, "Infanticide: When the Doctor's Orders Read Murder," he reported that charges of attempted murder filed against these parents and attending physician of the newborn Siamese twins brought the public's attention to a little known fact: "Infanticide by starvation and neglect is becoming more common in intensive-care nurseries – at the request of parents and by the order of physicians." Horan also reported that nurses are at risk of homicide charges, civil suits, and loss of license and reputation in the community while caught in the middle of the criminal activity.

According to Horan (1982), one professor of medical ethics participating in a discussion of the Danville case reported that *"most"* of his "colleagues in medicine, nursing, philosophy, theology, and ethics believed that the initial decision of doctors and family not to begin life support, even feeding and a sip of water, was justifiable in light of the jeopardy the birth presented to the family and the drawn-out suffering implied for the children" (p. 82). One nurse reported the Danville twins as having three legs, one with a half foot with seven toes, two legs sticking out of one side and one on the other.

Summary

Infanticide, or the killing of an infant, has occurred throughout the nation for centuries. Usually, infanticide is confined to handicapped infants with several anomalies or to abortion of unwanted children.

The first offense of infanticide was introduced into the Law of England and Wales in 1922 and amended in 1938. The act applied only to women and resulted in probably a lesser penalty in cases where there was a mental imbalance attributable to birth, with the verdict and sentencing by the judge. However, provisions for attempted infanticide were not approved until the Criminal Attempts Act of 1981. In addition, the Rehabilitation Act of 1973 prohibited discrimination of care for the handicapped.

Later, the Child Abuse Amendments of 1984 provided that all state child service agencies, health care facilities, and health care professionals develop procedures to ensure that medically indicated treatment, nutrition, general care, and social services as appropriate be provided to infants at risk with life-threatening congenital impairments. The Act also included special requirements for HHS to: publish guidelines for review of care provided to infants at risk, develop a resource directory, and determine effective means for providing financial support to meet the medical needs of at-risk infants. In 1973, the Supreme Court decision, Roe vs. Wade, legalized abortion. The Hyde Amendment in 1979 restricted funding for abortion to cases of rape or incest.

Despite legislation, ethics committees to assist in decision making for infants at risk, thoughts of health care professionals, right-to-life groups, or other individuals, infanticide continues to be a concern. Whether it is neonaticide (parents killing of an infant) or active euthanasia (hastening the infant's death), the question remains, "Is infanticide right or wrong?"

The government has the right to ensure that services and resources are available and enforce the laws. The parents have different viewpoints on infanticide. Some believe that they do have the right to make life or death decisions if there are multiple anomalies, stress on the family, financial burdens, and if the infant is only existing and cannot get better. Others cannot make decisions and request health care professionals to assist them.

Proponents of abortion think that termination of a fetus is not homicide; a woman has the right to control her body; no group or individual should force a woman to carry an unwanted pregnancy; and children have basic and constitutional rights of having parents who love and care for them and who can provide a safe environment. Anti-abortionists believe that even in the embryonic stage, the fetus is human life and that deliberate unjustified termination is homicide, especially abortion for choosing the sex of the baby.

Some believe that babies have a right to life and should not die because families cannot cope with them. Others think babies would prefer to die. Especially if life-support measures such as ventilators are required or if pain and suffering continue. Ethicists relate many reasons for infanticide such as all human beings are not persons unless the infant has minimal intelligence, a sense of future and past, can relate to others, has a balance between rationality and feeling, and has an IQ of at least 40. Others use formulas to establish quality of life.

Society also has a right to know the cost-benefit ratio of patients receiving Medicaid for maternity care and neonatal intensive care. The increasing demand on municipal services and higher taxes are also of grave concern.

Case reports of infanticide are found in the literature with regard to multiply-handicapped, Down's syndrome babies and low birth-weight infants who are withheld surgery, food, or other medical treatment. Some health care professionals appear to be involved in the decision-making process for life or death, and some are requesting ethics committees.

Physicians, nurses, and other health care professionals say that with all the new technical breakthroughs, it is going to be even more difficult to make the decisions on the life and death issue, because decisions may affect health care personnel who may suffer loss of employment and licensure.

Life and death decisions create an ethical dilemma for health care professionals – "to treat or not to treat" infants is a judgment to be made by someone. Unclear prognosis can affect everyone involved. Physicians and other health care workers do not want to prolong suffering of an incurable infant; yet they are dedicated to helping babies survive. However, the question on infanticide still remains a critical issue and an ethical dilemma: "Who has the right to pull the plug?"

Cited References

A new medical ethic. (1970). *California Medicine*, 67-68.

Annas, G. J. (1984). Public health and the law: The Baby Doe regulations – government intervention in neonatal rescue medicine. *American Journal of Public Health*, 74 (6): 618-620.

Annas, G. J. (1984). "Public health and the law": The case of Baby Jane Doe – child abuse or unlawful federal intervention? *American Journal of Public Health*, 74 (7): 727-729.

Benson, D. O. (1984). Court decision shouldn't be held up for abuse. *The Auburn Plainsman*, 93 (6): A-5.

Brown, S. S. (1989). Drawing women into prenatal care. *Perspectives*, 21 (2): 73-84.

Creighton, H. (1984). Law for the nurse manager: shall we choose life or let die. *Nursing Management*, 15 (8): 16-17.

Dilemmas in Practice: Withdrawing or withholding food and fluid. (1988). *American Journal of Nursing*, 88 (6): 797-801.

Fackelmann, K. A. (1986, June). *Medicine and Health. Perspectives*, 1-4.

Fletcher, J. (1980). Ethics and euthanasia. In D. J. Horan and D. Mall, eds., *Death, Dying, and Euthanasia*, p. 301. Frederick, MD: University Publications of America.

Fletcher, J. (1972). Indicators of humanhood: a tentative profile of man. *Hastings Center Report*, 3.

Horan, D. J. (1980). Euthanasia as a form of medical management. In *Death, Dying, and Euthanasia*, pp. 196-227.

Horan, D. J. (1982, January). Infanticide: when the doctor's orders read murder. *RN*: 75-86.

Institute of Medicine. (1985). *Preventing low birth weight*. Washington, D.C.: National Academy Press.

Jeffrey, R., Jeffrey, P., and Lyon, A. (1984). Female infanticide and amniocentesis. *Social Science Medicine*, 19 (11): 1207-12.

Kenny, A. M., Torres, A., Ditters, N., and Macies, J. (1986). Medicaid expenditures for maternity and newborn care in America. *Perspectives*, 18 (3): 103-10.

Manney, J. M., and Blattner, J. C. (1985). Infanticide: murder or mercy. *Journal of Christian Nursing*, 2 (3): 10-14.

McCormick, R. A. (1974). To save or let die: the dilemma of modern medicine. *Journal of the American Medical Association*, 229 (2): 172-76.

Murray, Thomas H. (1985). Why solutions continue to delude us. *Social Science Medicine*, 20 (11): 1103-07.

News: HHS stands by Baby Doe policy despite court's rulings on regulations. (1983, June). *American Journal of Nursing*, 851, 868-869.

Parker, E., and Good, F. (1981, March). Infanticide. *The Observer Magazine*, 237-43.

Paris, J. J., and McCormick, R. A. (1983). Saving defective infants: Options for life or death. *American*, 313-17.

Prescott, J. W. (1976, Spring). Abortion or the unwanted child: choice for a humanistic society. *Journal of Pediatric Psychology*, 62-67.

Robinson, M., Pakter, J., and Svigir, (1974). Medicaid coverage of abortions in New York City: Costs and benefits. *Family Planning Perspectives*, 6: 202-208.

Rue, V. M. (1985) Death by design of handicapped newborns: the family's role and response. *Issues in Law and Medicine*, 1 (3): 201-25.

Thomas, C. L., 15th ed. (1985). *Taber's cyclopedic medical dictionary*. Philadelphia, PA: F. A. Davis Company, p. 839.

Tooley, M. (1972). Abortion and infanticide. *Philosophy and Public Affairs*, 2 (1): 37-65.

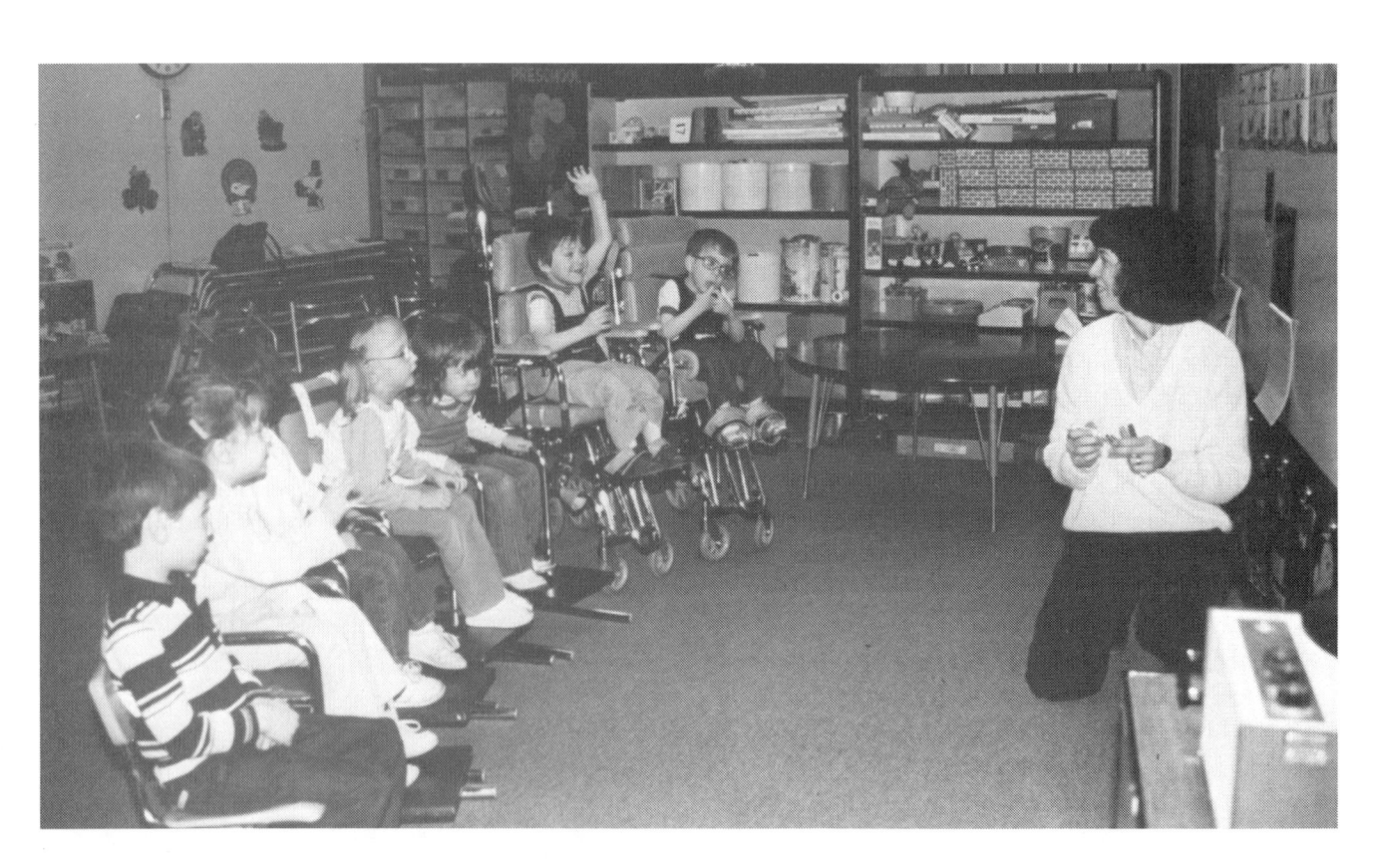

Baby with Congenital Abnormalities

A baby is born with numerous congenital abnormalities: no anal opening, a cleft palate and harelip, and the heart outside the body. The baby is a placid child who seems unaware of what is going on around her. The child's parents are on welfare and have several children.

- Would the parents of this child be likely to have the same degree of affection for this infant as they might have for their other children?

- What responsibility should some agency or the government have for this child? Should an agency (government) be expected to pay for this child's care if the parents are unable to provide for it?

- Could the mother have contributed to the baby's condition by doing such things during her pregnancy as eating improperly, wearing excessively tight clothes, smoking, drinking, or taking drugs?

- Could the father have contributed to the malformation by engaging in such activities before the conception as excessive drinking, using drugs, smoking, and sexual relationships with a variety of partners?

- If the baby's mother is a single parent, is her family responsible for assisting her? If so, in what way?

- Should the father of the baby and/or his parents be held accountable for the baby, and if so, to what degree?

- Suppose the mother is only fourteen years old. What rights does she have regarding what happens to her baby?

- If the father were the same age, would he have any rights or responsibilities?

- Suppose the baby resulted from a rape incident. What obligation does the mother have to the baby?

- If the parents of the child decide to allow the baby to die, does the physician or the hospital staff have any responsibility?

- If a person is old enough to have a baby, is that person mature enough to make a valid decision regarding the life of a child?

- At what age is someone mature enough to make decisions for other people?

- Is there any difference between aborting a fetus with abnormalities or letting a child die at or soon after birth?

- Suppose the decision is made to let the child die because of the poor quality of life it would have if it lived. Would it be more humane to give the child something to put it to sleep as compared to not feeding it and letting starve to death?

- Could this problem have been detected during the pregnancy? If so, should the physician have recommended some action prior to the delivery?

- Would you feel any differently if this were one of your siblings?

- If this were a child of a close friend or a neighbor, what action would you recommend?

- How would you feel if this were your child?

- What rights should a newborn child have, and who should look out for those rights?

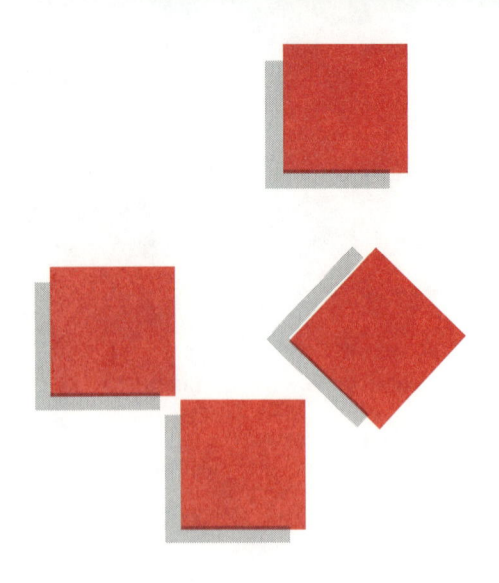

Photo Credits

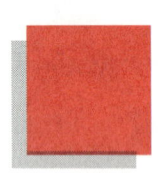

Roger Bean	61, 131, 140
The Bettmann Archive	62
Bristol-Myers	135
Barbara Caldwell	105
Campbell's Soup	80
CNS/Arturo Mari	51
Tony Freeman	96
Jim Gaffney	117
Ann Garvin	15
Hewlett Packard	121
Charles Hofer	102
Impact Communications	83
Thomas Jefferson School	131, 140
Journal Star / Al Harkrader	92
March of Dimes	82
Bob McElwee	11
National Kidney Foundation	34, 39, 41
North Wind Picture Archives	112
Proctor Community Hospital	52, 102
Liz Purcell	12, 29, 35, 37, 47, 93
Ross Laboratories	138
United Way	70
UPI / Bettman Newsphotos	46
The Upjohn Co.	25
Washington Post	27
Duane Zehr	84

Index

A

Abortion 133
    Medicaid funding 130
Abuse, fetal 130
Active euthanasia 116, 126
Advertising, subliminal 61
AIDS 26
Alcohol, and behavior 64
Alzheimer's disease 26
Ambulatory peritoneal dialysis 39
Amino acids, in gene splicing 20
Amniocentesis 68, 76, 82
Antibody 20
Artificial dialysis 34
Artificial insemination 44
    screening donors 81
Artificial kidney dialyzer 32
Autosomal recessive gene 76

B

Baby M Case 55
Behavior control 58
    role of government 63
Behavior modification 62
Behavioral practice 103
Beneficence 104
Bioengineer 20
Bioengineering process 21
Biological death 114
Biomedical Ethics 101,107
Biomedical research
    guidelines 104
Brain death 114
British eugenics movement 10
Brophy, Paul 118
Brown, Louise 46

C

Carrier screening 79
Catholic Church,
    in-vitro fertilization 51
Cellular death 114
Child Abuse Amendment of 1984 130
China, eugenics 10
Chorionic villi testing 87
Cloning 41, 44
Coma 110
Competency 116
Conroy, Clair 118
Consent 106
Consent, informed 44, 58
Continuous cyclic peritoneal dialysis 39
Contraception 8
Cost-benefit analysis,
    low birth-weight infants 135
Cost-containment issues,
    dialysis 36
Costs, dialysis 34
    handicapped children 134
in-vitro fertilization 49, 53
transplantation 93
Court cases, active euthanasia 121
    euthanasia 118
Cryopreservation 44, 50
Customs 70

D

Death 114
    infants 137
Decision making 71
    eugenics 15
Defects per live births 77
Deformed newborns 121
Dialysis, discontinuation 40
    kidney 94
    kidney, patient selection 32
DNA 20
    ligase 22
    probes 8, 12
    technology 22
Donors, artificial insemination
    screening 81
Down's syndrome 23, 26
Drug use 63
Duty-based approaches,
    decision making 71
Dying, costs 120

E

E. coli, in DNA research 23
Elderly, organ transplants 94
Embryos, transfer 44
    legal rights 50, 52
End-stage renal disease
    (ESRD) 32, 34
Ethical concerns, eugenics 13
    fetal research 70
    in-vitro fertilization 50
Ethics 70
    biomedical 107
    committees 13, 116, 136
    transplants 97
Eugenic manipulation,
    in-vitro fertilization 51
Eugenics 44
    hereditary traits 8
Euthanasia 110
    active vs. passive 119
Euthanasia, court cases 118
    Debbie 120
    international practices 122
Extrauterine surgery 69

F

Fecundity 8
Fertilization, in-vitro 8, 44
Fetal abuse 130
    alcohol syndrome 68
    blood sampling 83
    research 68
    screening 82
Fetology 68-69
alpha-Fetoprotein 68, 86
Fetoscopy 76, 83
Fetus 68
    rights 133
Fitness 15
Fletcher, Joseph 131
Follicular recruitment 44
Frozen embryos, legal rights 52
Funding issues, dialysis 34

G

Galactosemia 23
Galton, Francis 10
Gamete intrafallopian transfer
    (GIFT) 44
Gametes 8
Genes 20
    splicing 20
    therapy, uses 26
Genetics
    mass screening 76
    engineering 8, 12
    inferiority 12
    screening, populations 77
Genotypes 76
Gilbert, Ros 121

H

Handicapped children, costs 134
    infants, treatment decisions 131
Heart transplantation 92
Hemodialysis 32, 34, 38
Herbert, Clarence 118
Hereditary traits 16
    eugenics 8
Heredity, expenses 11
Heterozygote 76
Hippocratic oath 102
Home dialysis 37, 40
Human being, behavior control 58
    definition 132
    experimentation, scientific
        knowledge 100
    growth hormone (hGH) 24
    immune system 26
    subjects, protection 103
Human Tissue Fetal Transplant
    Research Panel 73
Humulin 24
Hypothyroidism screening 80

I

Identity tags, DNA 21
Immune response 20
Immunosuppressive drugs 90, 92

143

Individual freedom 17
Infant deaths 137
    euthanasia 134
Infanticide 126
    Act 128
    legislation 128
    male vs. female 134
Informed consent 44, 58
Interferon 20
Interleukin-2 26
International practices,
    euthanasia 122
In-vitro fertilization 44, 48
Irreversible coma 115

J

Jobes, Nancy 118
Justice 104

K

Kidney dialysis 94
    patient selection 32
Kidney transplantation 92

L

Laws 70
Legislation, infanticide 128
Life and death decisions 132
Life-support systems 97
Living wills 116
Lobotomies 62
Low birth-weight infants,
    cost-benefit analysis 135

M

Manipulation 58
Mass screening,
    for genetic disorders 76
Maternity care,
    patients and costs 135
Medicaid funding, abortion 130
Medical practice 103
Medicare reimbursement,
    transplants 94
Mental manipulation 60
Monoclonal antibodies 26
    technology 22
Morality 70
Morals 45

N

Negative eugenics 11
Neonatal intensive care 135
Neonaticide 126, 130
Neural tube defects 69
Newborns, deformed 121
    screening 80
Netherlands,
    guidelines for euthanasia 120
Nuremburg code 100, 103

O

Occupational settings,
    genetic screening 84
Oocyte recovery 43

Organ transplantation 90
    costs 93
    history 95

P

Passive euthanasia 116
    court cases 118
Patient selection,
    kidney dialysis 32
Peritoneal dialysis 32, 34, 39
Peritoneum 32
Persistent vegetative
    state 110, 115
Person, definition 132
Phenylketonuria 23
    screening 80
Philosophical perspective,
    eugenics 12
Physical manipulation 60
Placebo 100, 106
Plasmid 22
Political perspective, eugenics 11
Polymorphism 76
Poor patients,
    organ transplantation 94
Populations,
    for genetic screening 77
Positive eugenics 11
Practice 103
Premises, level of 71
Prenatal screening 8
President's Commissions for the
    Study of Ethical Problems in
    Medicine and Biomedical and
    Behavioral Research 12, 65
Principles, level of 71
Program planning,
    genetic screening 77
Protection, human subjects 103
Psychosurgery 58, 62
Psychotropic drugs 62
Psychotherapeutic Centers 62
Public Law 92-103
    dialysis 36
Public safety,
    recombinant DNA 24
Pull the plug decisions 97

Q

Quality of life formula 131
    issues, dialysis 38
    organ transplant 92
Quinlan, Karen Ann 118

R

Randomized clinical trials 106
Recombinant DNA 21
    products 24
    technology 22
Recreational drugs,
    and behavior 64
Rehabilitation Act 129
Renal function, dialysis 34
Research 103

fetal tissue 73
monitoring 106
standards 105
Restriction enzyme 121
Results-based approaches,
    decision making 71
Rights, embryo 50
    fetus 133
Rights-based approaches,
    decision making 71
Rules, level of 71

S

Scientific knowledge,
    human experimentation 100
Scientific perspective, eugenics 12
Screening, for carriers 79
    for genetic disorders 76
    newborns 80
    in occupational settings 84
    prenatal 8
Sex choice, role in infanticide 134
Sex-linked disease 45, 83
Sickle-cell anemia 80
Singapore, eugenics 10
Social problems, eugenics 11
Splicing genes 20
Standards of research 105
Subliminals 58
    advertising, in Mexico 60
    messages 60
Success rates,
    in-vitro fertilization 47
Supply and demand,
    organs for transplant 95
Surgical procedures in-utero 69
Surrogate mothers 44, 48

T

Tay-Sachs disease 79
Terminally ill 110
Test-tube babies 45
Tissue, fetal, research 73
Tissue plasminogen activator
    (TPA) 25
Tooley, Michael 131
Transplantation, of organs 90

U, V

Ultrasonography 68
Ultrasound imaging 82
United States,
    eugenics movement 10
Unwanted children 133
Uremia 32
Vegetative state 114
Viruses, in recombinant
    DNA techniques 28
Voluntary euthanasia 116

W, X, Y, Z

Whitehead, Mary Beth 55
Wrongful life 50
X-linked recessive 76
Zygmaniak, Lester 121